Cog
The

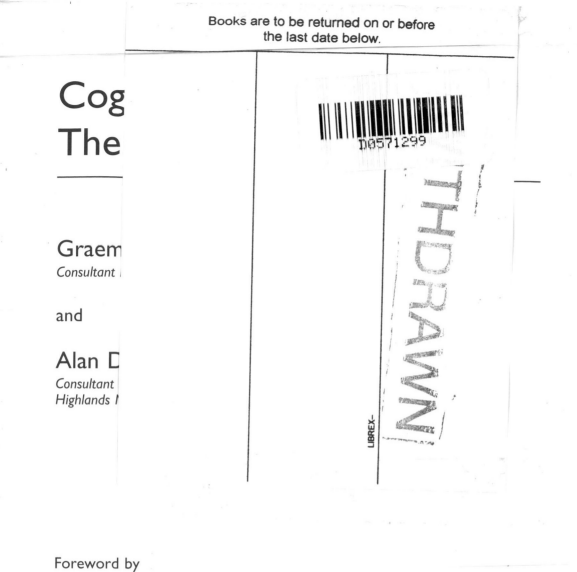

Graem

Consultant

and

Alan D

Consultant
Highlands

Foreword by
Anne Garland

Radcliffe

Oxford •

Radcliffe Publishing Ltd
18 Marcham Road
Abingdon
Oxon OX14 1AA
United Kingdom

www.radcliffe-oxford.com
Electronic catalogue and worldwide online ordering facility.

British Library Cataloguing in Publication Data

A catalogue record for this book is available from the British Library.

ISBN: 978 1 85775 603 6

Typeset by Anne Joshua & Associates, Oxford
Printed and bound by TJI Digital, Padstow, Cornwall

Contents

Foreword

This timely text by Whitfield and Davidson offers an excellent introduction to the basic theoretical principles and clinical interventions within the CBT model. It begins with an informative historical overview outlining the development of CBT practice as we know it today. This encompasses its origins in behaviourism, through learning theories to more recently developed cognitive models and concludes with a discussion of current cutting edge cognitive and behavioural interventions that have integrated research evidence from cognitive science into their treatment protocols.

The book is replete with concise definitions of commonly used terminology in psychotherapy as well as CBT, which lends a level of clarity and accessibility that gives the book ready appeal to a broad readership. This, alongside the book's emphasis on integrating CBT principles and practices into generic mental health and social care roles, means it will be of benefit to mental health nurses, social workers, occupational therapists, psychology assistants, as well as its target audience of psychiatrists in training. The contents are of relevance to any mental health professional working in both primary and secondary health and in social and voluntary sector care settings.

The book advocates the use of CBT interventions supported by research evidence for their effectiveness and provides a comprehensive guide to NICE recommendations for CBT interventions to be used in the treatment and management of mental health problems. This will be an indispensable resource for any mental health professional whose clinical governance standards stipulate that their clinical interventions with service users' treatment need to be informed by NICE recommendations.

The chapters in the book which cover the practical application of CBT in the treatment of mental health problems highlight with clarity the core clinical skills required to practice CBT safely and effectively, emphasising the importance of participating in CBT training and clinical supervision in order to develop and maintain robust CBT skills. The text makes clear and relevant links between CBT theory and clinical interventions, guiding the reader in a step-wise way through the disorder-specific CBT models for the treatment of mental health problems.

Overall this book makes an excellent contribution to the CBT literature. It will prove to be a valuable guide to those clinicians wishing to develop their CBT knowledge and skills and a useful resource in both personal and organisational libraries. It would be ideally referenced on the reading list of introductory CBT training courses and websites aiming to promote e-learning based CBT training initiatives within health and social care organisations. An accessible and informative text for novices to CBT.

Anne Garland
Consultant Nurse in Psychotherapy
Nottinghamshire Healthcare NHS Trust
January 2007

Preface

This introductory text has been written for beginners who need an overview of the cognitive behavioural therapy (CBT) approach. As such it is intended for postgraduate trainees in psychiatry, psychology, psychiatric nurses and interested general practitioners as well as undergraduate medical and nursing students. It has been written to complement *Dynamic Psychotherapy Explained* (2e) by Hughes and Riordan. As far as possible the two publications have been written in a similar style so that trainees who have used that publication will be familiar with the approach of this introduction to CBT. *Cognitive Behavioural Therapy Explained* attempts to describe the basic cognitive behavioural approach.

The book is written in three parts. Each part is made up of a number of chapters. Part 1 gives a general background to CBT. It includes a general description of the history of CBT, the theories that underpin the practice of CBT and the ways in which CBT principles can be delivered in psychiatric practice. It also outlines the current evidence base for CBT and associated UK practice guidelines. Part 2 outlines the practical aspects of undertaking CBT with a patient, including how to conceptualise a patient using CBT-informed formulations. It also describes some of the better-known cognitive and behavioural techniques. Part 3 concentrates on the different areas of mental disorder and how CBT practice is specifically delivered for these disorders. There is a brief overview of the major cognitive behavioural models that apply to each diagnostic area, followed by the major assessment questions and treatment approaches that are also specific to that diagnosis. Practical examples illustrate the processes involved and make the text more interesting and 'real'.

A short number of references for further reading are provided at the end of each chapter. It must be emphasised that these references are neither the most comprehensive nor necessarily the most up to date. They have been chosen because the authors believe them to be particularly useful in further illuminating the subject area for the target audience for this book. Postgraduate trainees in psychiatry and psychiatric nursing frequently have huge amounts of material to learn, therefore the emphasis within this book has been to present enough information that a trainee might usefully know for membership and postgraduate examinations without going into undue detail. If the student finds a subject particularly interesting, the further reading provided could deepen the knowledge base and interest as required.

This book was originally written out of necessity – namely as a text for juniors in psychiatry who need to know about CBT for their Royal College membership examinations. At the time that both of the current authors sat their own 'membership exams', there did not appear to be any texts that summarised the required information in a clear and basic fashion. *Cognitive Behavioural Therapy Explained* attempts to change this and indeed has been written mainly by compiling teaching notes that the authors have used with psychiatrists in training over a number of years. It is hoped that this experience of trainee psychiatrist supervision is apparent from the text. It is also hoped that the enthusiasm that the authors hold for psychological therapies and CBT in particular is apparent, and that this enthusiasm and interest can be imparted to practitioners who, quite understandably, may not use CBT as their predominant treatment modality.

Graeme Whitfield
Alan Davidson
January 2007

About the authors

Graeme Whitfield MB ChB, MSc, MRCPsych is a Consultant Psychiatrist in Psychotherapy (CBT) in Leicester. He is accredited with, and is a past governing board member of, the British Association for Behavioural and Cognitive Psychotherapies (BABCP).

Alan J W Davidson MB, ChB, MRCP, MRCPsych is a Consultant Psychiatrist working in both general adult psychiatry and psychotherapy (CBT) in the West of Scotland. He is also accredited with the BABCP.

Acknowledgements

We should like give special thanks to Chris Williams whose enthusiasm for CBT and vision of how it may be flexibly delivered has influenced both authors. We would also like to thank the psychiatric senior house officers in Leicester, Leeds and the West of Scotland who read through and gave helpful feedback from a trainee's point of view. Finally, we would like to thank Patricia Hughes and Dan Riordan for the book *Dynamic Psychotherapy Explained* (2e), which has been used as an invaluable teaching tool by both of us and was the inspiration for the creation of *Cognitive Behavioural Therapy Explained*.

Abbreviations

AN	anorexia nervosa
BABCP	British Association for Behavioural and Cognitive Psychotherapies
BAI	Beck Anxiety Inventory
BD	bipolar disorder
BDD	body dysmorphic disorder
BDI	Beck Depression Inventory
BED	binge-eating disorder
BMI	body mass index
BN	bulimia nervosa
BPD	borderline personality disorder
BT	behaviour therapy
CAT	cognitive analytic therapy
CBP	cognitive behavioural psychotherapy
CBT	cognitive behavioural therapy
CBT-BED	CBT focused on binge-eating disorder
CCBT	computerised cognitive behavioural therapy
CMHT	community mental health team
COPD	chronic obstructive pulmonary disease
CORE	clinical outcomes in routine evaluation
CPN	community psychiatric nurse
CTS-R	revised cognitive therapy scale
DAs	dysfunctional assumptions
DAS	Dysfunctional Attitude Scale
DBT	dialectical behaviour therapy
DSM	Diagnostic and Statistical Manual of Mental Disorders
DTR	Dysfunctional Thought Record
EE	expressed emotion
EMDR	eye movement desensitisation and reprocessing
EMS	early maladaptive schemas
ERP	exposure and response prevention
GAD	generalised anxiety disorder
GDG	Guideline Development Group
GE	graded exposure
GP	general practitioner
GPP	good practice points
ICD	International Classification of Diseases
ICS	interacting cognitive subsystems
IPSRT	interpersonal and social rhythm therapy
IPT	interpersonal therapy
NATs	negative automatic thoughts
NICE	National Institute for Health and Clinical Excellence

NIMH	National Institute of Mental Health
OCD	obsessive-compulsive disorder
PD	panic disorder
PI	psychodynamic interpersonal therapy
PTSD	post-traumatic stress disorder
RCT	randomised controlled trial
REBT	rational emotive behaviour therapy
SSRI	selective serotonin re-uptake inhibitors

Introduction

Psychological therapies are popular with clients. In this age when medicines offer real hope for most mental illnesses, population surveys still show that people frequently want to address mental health problems using talking treatments (Jorm *et al*, 1997). Unfortunately, psychological therapies are also expensive to deliver. Furthermore, there are too few cognitive behavioural therapy (CBT) therapists in the UK – approximately 1000 therapists are BABCP accredited for the whole nation (British Association for Behavioural and Cognitive Psychotherapies (BABCP) figures (updated regularly on BABCP website www.babcp.org.uk)). This situation may change over time with prominent political initiatives (Layard, 2006). Nevertheless, it is acknowledged by many, including the Royal College of Psychiatrists, that non-CBT therapists should have a good working knowledge of CBT, to be able to think within a cognitive behavioural framework, even if the majority of their work does not involve formal psychotherapy (Royal College of Psychiatrists, 2002).

Cognitive behavioural principles have been influential in the design and service delivery of many recent health-sector initiatives. Early-onset psychosis services, assertive outreach, and intensive home treatment teams all incorporate elements of cognitive behavioural thinking, even if it is primarily concentrated upon problem-solving skills and behavioural change. Some services integrate more formal cognitive behavioural therapy into their work. The role of professionals within these services is changing – roles that previously involved simply pre-scribing and monitoring of mental state are changing into roles that have a more explicit element of psychological therapy. Pressure to deliver this psychological therapeutic element comes not only from public opinion, but also from research. CBT, more so than any other model of psychological therapy, has been shown in research to be efficacious for a wide range of mental disorders. In the UK, the agency given the role of assessing that research base and then providing guidance to the NHS is the National Institute for Health and Clinical Excellence (NICE) at nice.org.uk. Their guidelines have consistently advocated psychological therapies (most frequently CBT) for a range of disorders. They have stated that CBT should be provided for many disorders within standard services (*see* Chapter 4 of this book).

Because of these changes, it is becoming imperative that psychiatrists, psychiatric nurses and general practitioners be knowledgeable of the cognitive behavioural approach. They need to know when to refer for CBT, who to refer and to be able to use cognitive behavioural principles within their daily work. A minority of psychiatrists will take more of a lead role to deliver CBT to more challenging patients, to teach it to juniors and to act as a 'product champion' in order to effect dissemination of skills to other practitioners (Whitfield *et al*, 2006). It was with this aim in mind that this book was written – not to produce cognitive behavioural psychotherapists *per se*, but to assist psychiatrists, psychiatric nurses and other mental health staff to know enough about the theory and practice of CBT to begin to incorporate aspects into their practice. It is also hoped that it will enthuse some to take an even greater interest in CBT and to encourage them to take up more formalised diploma- or masters'-level postgraduate training.

Further reading

- Jorm AF, Korten AE, Jacomb PA *et al.* (1997) Helpfulness of interventions for mental disorders: beliefs of health professionals compared with the general public. *British Journal of Psychiatry* **171**: 233–7.

Part 1

Background to cognitive behavioural therapy

Chapter 1

What is cognitive behavioural therapy?

Definition of psychotherapy • Definition of cognitive behavioural therapy •
Characteristics of all psychotherapies • Classification of the psychotherapies •
Cognitive behavioural therapy • Psychodynamic (psychoanalytic) psycho-
therapy • Interpersonal therapy • Counselling • Cognitive analytic therapy •
Family (systemic) therapy • Couples therapy and group therapy

Definition of psychotherapy

> Psychotherapy is the treatment of emotional, behavioural or per-
> sonality problems by psychological means.
>
> (Hughes, 1999, p. 34)

This definition is broad – it needs to be, psychotherapies are numerous and diverse.
Nevertheless, all psychotherapies have the general aim of improving general
functioning and/or symptoms. This chapter attempts to outline the general
features of cognitive behavioural therapy and to compare this form of therapy
with the other main forms of therapy commonly used in mental health services. It
does not describe in detail the other main forms of psychotherapy and the reader is
directed to *Dynamic Psychotherapy Explained* (Hughes and Riordan, 2006) for further
information on this form of therapy.

Definition of cognitive behavioural therapy

Aaron T. Beck defined cognitive therapy as:

> an active, directive, time-limited, structured approach used to treat a
> variety of psychiatric disorders.
>
> (Beck, *et al*, 1979, p. 3)

For the purpose of this book the terms cognitive behavioural psychotherapy,
cognitive behavioural therapy, and cognitive therapy will be used interchangeably.
The vast majority of therapists in this area would happily describe their therapy as
'cognitive behavioural therapy' (CBT) or 'cognitive behavioural psychotherapy'
(CBP).

Characteristics of all psychotherapies

- An intense, emotionally charged, *confiding relationship* with a helping person.
- A rationale which contains an *explanation* of the patient's distress and of the
  methods for its release.

- The provision of *new information* about the nature and origins of the patient's problems and of ways of dealing with them.
- The installation of *hope* in the patient that he can expect help from therapy.
- An opportunity for experiences of success during the course of therapy, and a consequent enhancement of the *sense of mastery.*
- The facilitation of *emotional arousal* in the patient (Frank, 1971).

Classification of the psychotherapies

The main forms of psychological therapy available include:

- cognitive behavioural therapy
- psychodynamic (psychoanalytic) psychotherapy
- interpersonal therapy (IPT)
- counselling
- cognitive analytic therapy (CAT)
- family therapy
- couples therapy
- group therapy.

Cognitive behavioural therapy

The Royal College of Psychiatrists defines CBT as:

> a way of talking about:
> - how you think about yourself, the world and other people
> - how what you do affects your thoughts and feelings.
>
> CBT can help you to change how you think ('Cognitive') and what you do ('Behaviour'). These changes can help you to feel better. Unlike some of the other talking treatments, it focuses on the 'here and now' problems and difficulties. Instead of focusing on the causes of your distress or symptoms in the past, it looks for ways to improve your state of mind now.
>
> (Royal College of Psychiatrists, 2005, p. 1)

Cognitive behavioural therapy, and behavioural therapy before it, has always emphasised the fact that the therapist is *active* and *directive*. This means that the therapist actively steers the direction of the therapy and, rather than necessarily allowing the client to decide the content of the sessions, will suggest the tasks that need to be tackled within the sessions and the strategies that should be used.

Trust between the client and the therapist is as important in cognitive and behavioural therapy as it is in any other form of psychological therapy (Waddington, 2002). There is an emphasis on the client and the therapist working together to form a *'therapeutic alliance'*. In the spirit of this alliance, both the therapist and client may suggest items that they would like to discuss within each session (agreed upon at the beginning of the session). Therefore, the content of each session is *planned and structured* according to an agreed *session agenda*. This very much marks CBT out as different from other less directive and less structured forms of therapy, such as psychodynamic therapy and most counselling practice. The agenda will be influenced by the general direction of therapy that has been taken from the client's and therapist's *shared understanding of the problem*. This shared understanding should extend to a *written formulation* that is referred to repeatedly throughout therapy to direct, structure, and assess the impact of therapy (Persons, 1989). The formulation will also generate a number of specific goals that the client and the therapist agree upon at the beginning of therapy. This explicit *goal setting* is also more apparent in CBT relative to most other forms of psychological therapy (Persons, 1989). At the time that Beck was initially formulating the CBT approach in the 1960s and 70s most therapy in the UK was psychodynamic in orientation, and much of that was open-ended, i.e. not time limited. Today, due to constraints of time and resources, psychodynamic therapy is more often 'brief' in nature, so that it also has tended to become *time limited* (in common with CBT). This means that an agreed *number of sessions will be decided upon at the beginning of the course of therapy*. Similarly, counselling, which within the UK health service is most often provided within primary care, is now usually time limited.

Cognitive behavioural therapy is derived from models devised and evaluated within the academic discipline of *behavioural and cognitive psychology*. This has contributed to the current significant *evidence base* that supports the efficacy of cognitive behavioural therapy for a range of disorders. This evidence base is currently less developed in most other forms of psychological therapy. Another principle of cognitive behavioural therapy that marks it out as different from other models is the emphasis placed on 'putting into practice' the principles that have been learned in-session. This is often described as *'homework'*. Homework also allows for *testing out hypotheses* (note again the 'scientific model'), to be analysed at the next session. Integral to testing is the principle and the practice of measurement, and, indeed, the agreement to look only at the *'measurable'*. This may include the measurement of the extent that a belief is held and of behaviours that are carried out. Indeed, the effectiveness of strategies employed within therapy are constantly *monitored and evaluated* and changed depending on these results. This measurement includes the more extensive use of *rating scales* than traditionally has been the case for other therapies. The unconscious is not measurable, and this is one reason why Aaron T. Beck did not use the concept in his original theories. Similarly, the practice of CBT emphasises events in the *'here and now'*, rather than extensive exploration of the client's background (and particularly their childhood) as is the case for psychodynamic psychotherapy. The purposeful recreation of features of past relationships between the client and the therapist is not a feature of CBT. In contrast such 'transferential relationships' and the interpretation of unconscious motives is a major part of psychodynamic psychotherapy.

The number of sessions generally assigned to the therapy varies depending upon factors such as the disorder that is being treated. For example, panic disorder may be appropriately treated in 12 sessions (Wells, 1997), whereas CBT for personality problems takes significantly longer – often 12–24 months (Linehan, 1993). Herein lies another important difference between cognitive behavioural therapy and other models such as psychodynamic psychotherapy. That is that the CBT techniques used for one disorder may be quite significantly different from those techniques used for other disorders. This is less likely to be the case, particularly in psychodynamic therapy. The reason for this specific CBT approach to different disorders relates to the *'cognitive content specificity hypothesis'* (Beck *et al*, 1985). In essence this states that there are characteristic themes of thinking with associated cognitive errors or distortions associated with each disorder. Therefore, the major theme noted by Beck in depression was of *loss*, and in anxiety disorders it was of *threat*. This is important because, by extension, the models and the techniques used *differ significantly depending on the disorder* treated. Therefore, the CBT model and techniques used in treating depression may not be appropriately used in the treatment of eating disorders or post-traumatic stress disorder (PTSD). Indeed, the abbreviations sometimes used to describe the CBT for the disorders may include the abbreviation for that disorder to emphasise the differences (e.g. CBT-BN [bulimia nervosa] as described in the NICE guidelines CG9 2004 (*Eating Disorders*) for the treatment of bulimia). This is also why this book categorises the models of therapy and the treatment approaches into the disorders. This requirement would not be so apparent in other models of therapy such as psychodynamic therapy, where the overarching model and techniques differ less between the specific illness areas.

Psychodynamic (psychoanalytic) psychotherapy

Psychodynamic psychotherapy is also called psychoanalytic psychotherapy (*see* Hughes and Riordan, 2006) and has its origins in the theories of *Sigmund Freud*. It is one of the most widely practised forms of psychological therapy in the UK. It is acknowledged as having a clearer role in complex presentations where childhood experiences link with the current presentations, and where the need to find *personal meaning* from past events is important. Personality disorder is one area where psychodynamic models are often applied, including in *therapeutic communities*, which are usually run along psychodynamic principles. This form of therapy explores the influence of past events on current functioning and is described as an '*exploratory*' or '*insight-directed*' form of therapy.

Unlike the 'therapeutic alliance' in cognitive behavioural therapy, the working relationship in psychodynamic therapy attempts to recreate features of previous relationships. Known as '*transference*', the client begins to relate towards the therapist in a way that they may have done towards other important people in their past or current life. The relationship between the client and therapist is then analysed to explore the client's conscious and unconscious expectations and models of the world (Hughes and Riordan, 2006). The relationship is therefore described as a necessary '*active part of treatment*' in this form of therapy, in a way that it is not in other models of therapy. Transference should only be encouraged when it is safe to do so. For example, some patients should not be offered this form of therapy when they have poor '*ego strength*', that is they would feel overwhelmed and have a tendency to self-harming behaviour when faced with a recreation of some traumatic previous relationship. Others find it difficult to understand the intensity of the transference and the fact that it is only a recreation. They are likely to 'act-out' towards the therapist, e.g. in terms of threats of violence and stalking.

There is a general emphasis in psychodynamic therapy on *unconscious motivations* of the client and the effect this has on relationships. The therapist seeks to *interpret* behaviours, thoughts, and even dreams as evidence of that which is occurring in the patient's unconscious. The relationship is supportive, but there is usually not an active and direct problem-solving approach as there often is in both counselling and cognitive behavioural approaches. There is more of an emphasis on understanding and describing the patient's 'state of mind' and the influences working upon this from the patient's earlier, particularly childhood, life. How they then choose to use that information is left open to the patient, although the therapist will often explore other potential more useful ways of behaving and relating to others. In the UK, psychodynamic therapy is more often offered to people who are distressed but who may *not have a formal Axis I (DSM-IV, Diagnostic and Statistical Manual of Mental Disorders) diagnostic label* than is the case with cognitive behavioural therapy. The latter is more commonly applied to illness areas, such as for clients referred with clear-cut depression or PTSD.

Interpersonal therapy

Interpersonal therapy (IPT) was initially used as a treatment for depression, although it has since been applied to other problem areas such as eating disorders. In common with cognitive behavioural therapy, it is a brief form of therapy – approximately 15 sessions – and also tends to work in the 'here and now' rather than concentrating on the origins of the symptoms in the patient's past. The therapist is 'active', and the transference is not the vehicle of change that it is in psychodynamic therapy. However, in common with psychodynamic therapy it has a strong emphasis on relationships with others and the effect that patterns of relationships have on the presenting symptoms.

Counselling

The term 'counselling' refers to a broad range of psychological treatments. In its most frequently used meaning it refers to a supportive and non-directive form of talking treatment otherwise known as '*Rogerian*' counselling. *Non-judgemental listening* is offered, where 'space' is given for the patient to express their thoughts about events. Often an active *problem-solving approach* is taken, and the therapist may also use their own experiences to guide the patient towards alternative ways of viewing a situation or changing behaviours. This form of therapy is not 'exploratory' in that it does not attempt to look in depth into previous experiences and relate them to current functioning. For this reason it is generally less likely to cause significant distress compared to psychodynamic therapy in some patients. Counselling tends to concentrate upon finding *coping strategies* that the patient has already used, and strengthening these by 'playing to the patient's own strengths'. Novel strategies are also tried out, and the patient is *encouraged and supported* throughout their endeavours by the counsellor. Once again, transference does not tend to be an active part of the therapeutic process. A caveat to this is the fact that counselling does include other models including 'dynamic counsellors', and 'cognitive behavioural counsellors'. The use of these models within counselling blurs even more the distinction between what constitutes psychotherapy and what constitutes counselling. In the UK, counselling is particularly common in:

- *primary care*: where a counsellor is sometimes referred to as the 'practice counsellor'. They deal with milder presentations, and tend to refer on those with resistant, recurrent and more complex presentations

- *clinics for certain physical illnesses*: these include HIV, and coronary care, and increasingly form an important part of the services offered for the management of chronic illnesses such as asthma and diabetes
- *the support of people struggling to deal with a life crisis*: this includes grief counselling to navigate people through the grief process
- *private practice*: in this capacity, the term 'counsellor' has been controversial in that it does not confer necessary requirements for training or even practice.

Cognitive analytic therapy (CAT)

This form of therapy can also be delivered either individually, in couples or in groups (see Ryle, 1995). In common with CBT the number of sessions received by the patient is predetermined and agreed upon at the beginning of the treatment. Most commonly it is 16 sessions, but it varies from 4 to 24 sessions (*see* http:www.acat.me.uk/catintroduction.php). The therapy emphasises 'reformulation', 'recognition' and 'revision'. It integrates a number of background theories including psychoanalysis and cognitive behavioural approaches as its name suggests, but also Kelly's 'Personal Construct' theory and developmental psychology. In the UK it is delivered within some specialised units as well as by CAT therapists who work alongside other therapists in general units. In common with CBT the initial written diagrammatic formulation is a key part of therapy. CAT also makes use of 'goodbye letters', which are a personalised summary of the situation and the treatment given to the patient by the therapist at the end of the therapy.

Family (systemic) therapy

There are a number of 'schools' of family therapy, although in the UK at least, the term 'family therapy' is often used interchangeably with the name of one of these schools – 'systemic therapy'. The emphasis in family therapy is on the effect of parts of the family unit on other parts. Sometimes, only one family member will be presented as 'the problem', whereas the problem may be viewed as the relationships within the family as a whole. For example, a child may be presented with behaviour difficulties, while it becomes apparent that there are few boundaries laid down within the family as a result of a lack of emotional connectivity between the parents. Other forms of family therapy do exist, including cognitive behavioural family therapy. In general, family therapy services are found within services for children and families – mainly where the child is the 'presenting problem'. As such, it tends to be predominantly used with childhood and adolescent mental health problems such as behavioural problems, childhood depression and eating disorders, where the child or adolescent remains part of their original family unit. Where the child is less bound up with their family of origin – such as when they have moved out and have become more emotionally independent, then family therapy is less likely to be offered, and individual therapy is seen as more appropriate. In the treatment of patients with schizophrenia, family therapy is used to help family members reduce interpersonal stress. Interpersonal stress has been clearly shown to exacerbate psychotic symptoms (Vaughn and Leff, 1976).

Table 1.1 Summary of the major similarities and differences between cognitive behavioural therapy, dynamic psychotherapy and 'Rogerian' counselling

	Cognitive behavioural therapy	Dynamic psychotherapy	'Rogerian' counselling
Requires a trusting and confiding therapeutic relationship	Yes	Yes	Yes
Therapeutic relationship is the main 'vehicle for change'	No	Yes	No
Concentrates on earlier origins of problems	No	Yes	No
Concentrates on difficulties in the 'here and now'	Yes	No	May do
Is non-directive	No	Varies	Yes
Transference is a major part of therapy	No	Yes	No
Seeks to interpret 'unconscious motivations'	No	Yes	No
Emphasis is on direct problem solving	May be	No	Yes
Has a formulation to guide therapy	Yes	Yes	No
Homework is a major aspect	Yes	No	No
Is time limited	Yes	Sometimes	Usually
Is highly structured	Yes	No	No
Works to a session agenda	Yes	No	No
Uses experiments/data collection from the environment	Yes	No	No

The major differences between the three main forms of psychological therapy carried out in the UK (cognitive behavioural, psychodynamic, and counselling) are summarised in Table 1.1.

Couples therapy and group therapy

A detailed description of therapy in these formats is outside of the remit of this book. However, it is important to point out that psychotherapy from many different models can be delivered to both couples and to groups. For example, both psychodynamic psychotherapy and CBT are routinely delivered in groups although the emphasis of 'the group' is different. In some psychodynamic approaches the group dynamics are interpreted so that the emphasis is on 'analysis through and of the group'. More commonly in CBT the group is viewed more as a group of individuals who work together to learn and put into action the techniques in order to reduce symptoms and improve function. The situations within groups are, however, invariably more complex than that and Yalom (1975) summarises the curative factors that can occur in groups including catharsis, guidance and the use of imitation of one group member by another. Groups can also be very useful as a normalising experience where people see that their own experience is not unique, and therefore not so stigmatising.

MAIN POINTS

- A wide range of psychological therapy models are provided within the NHS. Three of the most common models are: CBT, psychodynamic psychotherapy and 'Rogerian' counselling. Family therapy is also available primarily within 'child and family' mental health services.
- There are differences between the models, but also commonalities. The latter have been described by Jerome Frank and include the need for a 'confiding relationship' and the 'instillation of hope'.
- CBT is an active, structured and time-limited form of therapy working primarily on problems in the 'here and now'.
- There are significant differences between the content of CBT provided for different forms of illness. This is in part due to the 'cognitive-content specificity hypothesis'.
- Psychodynamic psychotherapy is a form of 'exploratory' or 'insight-orientated' therapy. There is an emphasis within this therapy of finding 'personal meaning' from past (particularly childhood) events. Transference is an important part of therapy.
- 'Rogerian' counselling offers 'non-judgemental listening'. It concentrates upon offering support, encouragement and the role of coping strategies.
- There are different models of family therapy – including 'systemic' and 'cognitive behavioural'. Family therapy, particularly 'systemic family therapy', is interested in the influence of family relationships on the individual's 'presenting problem'.

Further reading

- Brown D and Pedder J (1979) *Introduction to Psychotherapy*. London: Tavistock Publications.
- Hughes P and Riordan D (2006) *Dynamic Psychotherapy Explained* (2e). Oxford: Radcliffe Publishing.

Chapter 2

Theoretical development of cognitive behavioural therapy

Theories of learning • Application of learning theories • Beck's model of depression • Rational emotive behavioural therapy • Further development of behavioural approaches • Application to new disorders • Closer links with cognitive psychology • Future directions

Theories of learning

Behaviour therapy emerged from theories of learning and their application. The two main theories of learning to know are classical conditioning and operant conditioning. These are summarised in Figures 2.1 and 2.2. *Classical conditioning* (based on the work of Pavlov and his dog!) relates to automatic responses that the animal (or person) makes in response to a stimulus. It is where an *unconditioned stimulus* such as a food becomes linked (paired) to another neutral stimulus such as a sound (e.g. a bell). Normally, the food would elicit an *unconditioned response* (e.g. salivation), and the sound of the bell ordinarily would not. With repeated pairings of the food and the sound, the animal salivates even when the sound (but no food) is presented. The sound has now become the *conditioned stimulus* and the salivation the *conditioned response*. The animal has been *conditioned* to respond to the sound by salivating.

The principles behind *operant conditioning* were described by Thorndike in his 'Law of Effect', and then extended by Skinner (1950). Unlike the salivation of Pavlov's dog, it involves conscious (i.e. non-automatic) learning. Operant conditioning involves a conscious change in behaviour that the animal or person makes in order to achieve a desired outcome. Quite simply it involves:

Stimulus → Response → Reward or punishment.

For example, at 9 am (the STIMULUS), you are required to be at work (the RESPONSE), and for doing your work you will be paid money (the REWARD).

When a given behaviour is followed by consequences, then the animal or person *learns* to either increase or decrease that behaviour (depending on whether the consequences are good or bad for it). Put another way, that response or behaviour becomes 'reinforced'. In essence, the consequences can be categorised into one of four types or *'contingencies of reinforcement'* (*see* Table 2.1). The consequences can be pleasant – so that the animal or person is *'rewarded'* – also known as *positive*

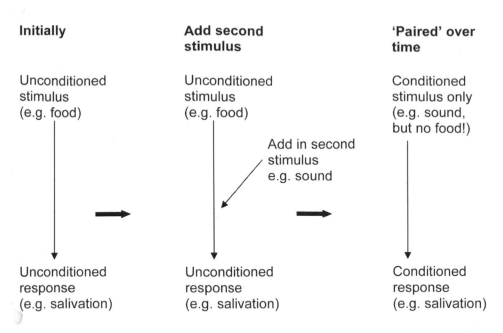

Figure 2.1 Classical conditioning: Pavlov's dog developed a conditioned response (salivating) to the stimulus of sound alone.

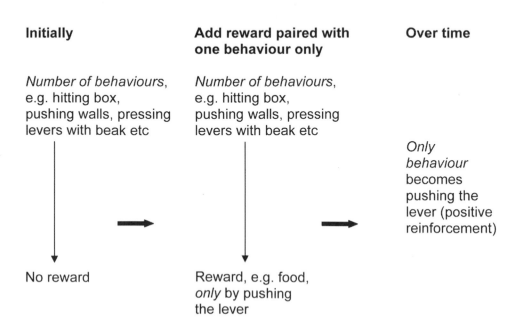

Figure 2.2 Operant conditioning: Skinner's animals learned that a behaviour would elicit a consequence that influenced (reinforced) how often they carried out that behaviour (the example given is positive reinforcement).

reinforcement. Note that *reward* was not a term preferred by Skinner himself. Alternatively, the consequences can be unpleasant – so that the animal or person is *'punished'*. This obviously reduces the likelihood that the person or animal will carry out that behaviour again. Less frequently seen are the other two types of consequence that comprise operant conditioning. One is where the potential pleasant consequence is taken away after the response – sometimes known as 'omission' or 'frustrative non-reward'. Finally, a potentially unpleasant consequence can also be taken away after the response, referred to as 'negative reinforcement'. Predictably, both reward and negative reinforcement lead to an increase in the resulting behaviour, while punishment and frustrative non-reward lead to a decrease in the resulting behaviour. At first, reading this can be difficult to grasp so its always best to think of examples – if we take a child and give a *reward*, such as 30 minutes on the internet for completing his or her homework, then this will increase the likelihood that the response (completing the homework) will be completed again. If they are scolded for failing to look after their younger sibling while studying, by a parent who does not value homework, then the child has been *punished* and will be less likely to do the homework another night. If the child is expecting a reward such as time on the internet, and this fails to happen after completing the work, then this is an example of *'frustrative non-reward'*, and once again the child is less likely to do the work another night. Finally, if the child is carrying out (or expecting to have to carry out) an unpleasant task such as cleaning their room, and their parent offers to do this for them if they do their homework, then this would be an example of *negative reinforcement* – the removal of an unpleasant stimulus. Importantly though, if a behaviour is to be reinforced it must be *linked closely in time* with the consequences – praising a child will only be effective in shaping behaviour if the praise occurs very soon after the given behaviour. This is a common failing in interventions that attempt to influence behaviours through feedback.

Therefore, when a behaviour (response) is reinforced, it alters the likelihood that that behaviour will be repeated. However, more commonly, any given behaviour will not have a given consequence *every* time it is carried out. A child may be scolded for being loud but rather than the parent's response occurring with every scream from the child, parents tend to respond only 'every so often'. Skinner termed this *'partial reinforcement'* in contrast to those behaviours that always elicit a response – *'continuous reinforcement'*. Perhaps surprisingly, once behaviour has been reinforced, it is harder to break that link (called *'extinction'*), if the behaviour has been acquired though partial rather than continuous reinforcement. Therefore, where a child's good behaviour has been positively reinforced intermittently by the

Table 2.1 The four categories or 'contingencies' of reinforcement

	Consequences **added**	Consequences **taken away**
Positive consequences	Positive reinforcement (reward)	Frustrative non-reward (omission)
Negative consequences	Punishment	Negative reinforcement

occasional reward, the good behaviour is more likely to continue even when the rewards stop, compared to a situation where good behaviour is always rewarded, but then suddenly stops being rewarded.

Application of learning theories

Enthusiasm for these learning theories encouraged by animal experiments led to new practical applications. One of the major applications of operant conditioning within psychiatry was the use of 'token economies' (Ayllon and Azrin, 1968). This approach was mainly used on psychiatric wards with patients with chronic schizophrenia. In this technique, desired behaviours, for example undertaking personal hygiene, are reinforced by the award of tokens which can be exchanged later, most frequently for items from the hospital shop. Although successful, operant conditioning was probably only one factor within the token economy system that caused the final 'observed behaviours'.

Potential connections were made between classical conditioning and the formation of phobias (Watson, 1930). Thus, a person stung in childhood can develop a phobia to wasps. Indeed, through a process of 'generalisation' they may develop a phobia to all flying insects. More recently, the importance of operant conditioning in the maintenance of phobias has been acknowledged. One way in which this regularly occurs is though avoidance – phobics tell themselves that the only reason that they are safe is because they escaped or avoided a fearful situation – an example of negative reinforcement. The stimulus becomes associated with the emotion of fear by classical conditioning, and the avoidant response then becomes reinforced. Most treatments for phobias that developed use the principle of 'habituation', whereby the organism becomes acclimatised slowly to the feared situation. For example, Wolpe (1961) introduced the concept of 'systematic desensitisation', whereby patients were gradually exposed to the feared stimuli while undergoing relaxation (he suggested that relaxation and fear could not co-exist). More recently the technique known as 'graded exposure in vivo' has become more commonly used for a range of anxiety disorders. It similarly depends on the principle of habituation, but generally does not incorporate relaxation. Rather, it aims to allow the person to fully experience the fear so that habituation to that fear can occur unimpeded.

Cognitions neglected

Although the behavioural approach was considered to be successful at both explaining and treating anxiety problems, there was less confidence that it was successful as a treatment for depression (Rachman, 1997). There was a growing realisation that the role of the client's thoughts or perception of a situation had an impact, as well as simply the stimulus and the resulting behaviours. *Bandura's* views on 'observational or social learning' (Bandura, 1977a) had an impact, proposing that cognitive factors played a part in learning. He stated that we do not learn simply by the effects that the environment has on us but also vicariously by observation of the behaviour of others. If we observe that someone else has success using a technique or tool, then we ourselves are likely to have learned that it is wise to do the same. Likewise, the degree to which the person perceived himself or herself capable of carrying out the behaviour (a cognitive judgement called *self-efficacy* by Bandura, 1977b) impacted upon whether the behaviour would occur or not. These factors have been incorporated into the approaches used by professionals, and into the treatment of phobias in particular. The therapist 'models' the feared behaviour (e.g. touching the spider), so that the patient learns that it is safe to do so. Similarly, patients are motivated through all CBT interventions, using the therapeutic relationship – thus encouraging self-efficacy so that the patient will be more willing to try things out.

It was fortuitous that it was during this period in the 1960s and 1970s that Aaron T. Beck was developing his 'cognitive therapy' for depression, fortuitous both that the emphasis was on thinking and that the subject was a condition that was proving difficult to treat – depression.

Beck's model of depression

Beck (1976, 1979) proposed that thoughts (cognitions) were not only a symptom of depression but, importantly, that they played a critical part in maintaining the depression. This differed in emphasis from earlier behavioural theories that had proposed that behaviours dictated outcome. Beck observed that patients with depression expressed characteristically negative views of themselves, the world and the future. He called this the *'negative cognitive triad'* of depression. In an attempt to explain these characteristically negative cognitions Beck proposed a model that separated out the thoughts of the individual into different 'levels' (*see* Figure 2.3). The most superficial layer of cognitions is the 'automatic thoughts'. This is the stream of thoughts that pass into our consciousness throughout the day – almost the 'background hiss' of thoughts! They usually relate to mundane events, but occasionally they have a content that evokes a significant emotion. Examples probably run to infinity, but would include thoughts such as 'it's midnight – I should go to bed', 'what shall I eat for breakfast?', 'I don't think that traffic light is going to stay green', etc. Beck proposed that at a deeper level we all have *rules or assumptions* that we hold about the world. These relate to a wide variety of issues that have been forged by our life experiences. Examples may include: 'if you work hard then you will be rewarded in the end', and: 'if you're slim then you're more likely to meet a partner'. Beck proposed that those who are prone to depression or who are depressed have a number of unhelpful rules that influence minute-to-minute thinking, producing automatic thoughts with a depressive content. He called these unhelpful rules *'dysfunctional assumptions'* (often shortened to DAs), and he called the resulting automatic thoughts with a depressive content *'negative automatic thoughts'* (often shortened to NATs). Examples of DAs in depression might be 'if I don't fit in then I'll be rejected', or 'if I don't have a job then I'm worthless', or 'I must always get good marks'. They can also relate to others: 'if you give others the chance they will use you'. Note that assumptions are usually 'if . . . then' statements, or include the words 'should', 'have to', 'must', etc. The resulting NATs from the rule 'if I don't have a job then I'm worthless' may include: 'I should not be off work'; 'Jim's a better bloke than I am – he's got a job'; 'my family think I'm a right waste of space'. It can be seen how such thoughts could cause the depressed person's mood to stay depressed! It is important to note that because automatic thoughts are always with us we do not generally question whether they are biased or problematic – we all have thoughts, but we rarely question their accuracy.

Finally, Beck proposed that at the deepest layer of cognition we hold quite rigid unconditional beliefs about ourselves, the world and others. These are termed *'schemas'* or *'core beliefs'*. In the example shown in Figure 2.3 the individual thinks that she is defective. Core beliefs can be positive but those that have a negative theme were proposed by Beck to be 'activated' in depression. These beliefs are expressed in short, unconditional terms such as 'I'm defective', or 'I'm unlovable',

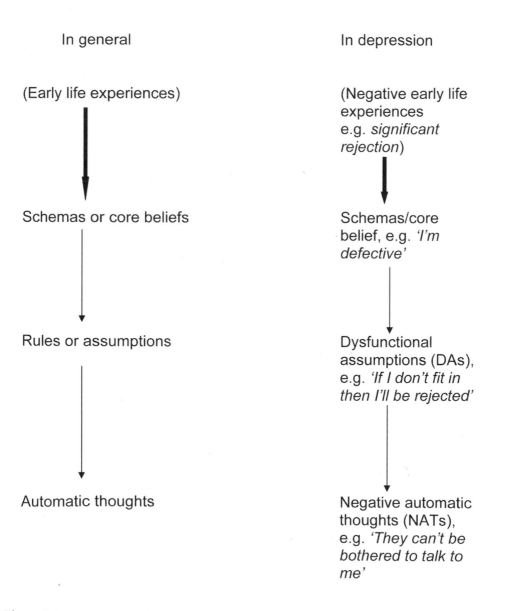

In general

(Early life experiences)

Schemas or core beliefs

Rules or assumptions

Automatic thoughts

In depression

(Negative early life experiences e.g. *significant rejection*)

Schemas/core belief, e.g. *'I'm defective'*

Dysfunctional assumptions (DAs), e.g. *'If I don't fit in then I'll be rejected'*

Negative automatic thoughts (NATs), e.g. *'They can't be bothered to talk to me'*

Figure 2.3 Beck's levels of cognition both generally and their proposed form in depression (*with example in italics*).

Table 2.2 Cognitive distortions in depression (Beck *et al*, 1979)

Cognitive distortion	Description of the distortion
1 Arbitrary inference	Basing a conclusion on inadequate evidence (or even on evidence that does not support the conclusion)
2 Selective abstraction	Taking a small amount of information and ignoring the 'wider picture' of information that is available. Conclusions are drawn only on that small amount of information
3 Overgeneralisation	Making up a rule based on a small number of incidents and then applying this rule to unrelated situations
4 Magnification and minimisation	Making an event greater in significance or lesser in significance than the evidence suggests is the case
5 Personalisation	Tendency of the person to unreasonably believe that events relate to himself or herself when they do not or they do so only to a small degree
6 Absolutistic or dichotomous thinking	Tendency to describe things in a very extreme way without 'shades of grey' – something is either *totally* great, or *totally* terrible

or 'I'm vulnerable'. Some may believe 'the world is dangerous', 'people are selfish' or even 'people are kind'. Beck hypothesised that we all hold core beliefs, that they have their origins in our early life experiences (although they can be altered to some extent by later experiences), and that their content shapes the development of our assumptions, and through them our automatic thoughts.

It is important to say that many of us have negative core beliefs, and all of us will have some DAs and NATs. Beck merely stated that in depression they are more prominent, and that their effects are to maintain the low mood.

Beck also stated that there are predictable processes by which NATs seemed to be formed in depression. He called these '*cognitive distortions*'. They are listed in Table 2.2. In practice there is overlap between the categories; some thoughts could be described as examples of more than one type of distortion. Furthermore, different people tend to use one or more of the distortions more than the others. For example, some depressed patients minimise the good in situations, while others characteristically can be observed repeatedly 'personalising' in their interactions with others. Much will relate to the content of the individual's schemas and to the environmental stressors that are challenging them. When the theme of the stressors has a particularly poignant significance for the individual, such as exams for someone who has a schema that they are 'inferior' and have to prove their worth, then the chances of illness increase:

> Demanding and unrealistic assumptions and rules are the fuel of auto-matic thoughts. Individuals who believe that they should be perfect or

they are failures may do fine until they experience a setback in their accomplishments. This setback will trigger a flood of negative thoughts (e.g., 'I always fail' or 'I'll amount to nothing') and activate the underlying schema (e.g., 'I'm a loser').

(Leahy, 2003, p. 333)

Beck noted that the theme of the activated schemas and the NATs varied to some extent, in a predictable way, between the disorders. The predominant theme in depression is loss and in anxiety it is threat.

Rational emotive behavioural therapy

Beck was not the only clinician to have noted the important role that thinking played in depression. Albert Ellis (1962) also put forward a form of therapy called rational emotive therapy (RET). He viewed irrational beliefs as a major cause of emotional disturbance and thought that these beliefs should be monitored and quite forcefully challenged. This then has many similarities to the 'Beckian' form of therapy. Another commonality is that it uses behavioural techniques. To respect this fact, the term 'RET' has extended to 'REBT', with the 'B' standing for 'behavioural'. There is a British Association of REBT that continues to have links with the lead organisation of CBT in Britain, the BABCP. Key differences between REBT and CBT include some of the more specific techniques used as well as the fact that REBT has a philosophical basis that emphasises concepts such as tolerance and social interest. Furthermore, REBT has not developed the evidence base that now supports the practice of cognitive behavioural therapy. As a form of therapy, REBT is much less frequently practised in the UK than CBT.

Further development of behavioural approaches

More recent years have continued to see the development of behavioural approaches in psychological medicine. Among many notable developments stands the work of Lewinsohn *et al* (1986). These workers hypothesised that depression was caused by a *deficiency of rewards* from repetitive and unrewarding surroundings (such as repetitive boring work). Behavioural therapy correspondingly recommended behavioural changes that increased the number of rewards gained from day-to-day living. This approach has continued within cognitive behavioural therapy in the form of 'activity scheduling' described further in Chapter 6 and 7. The emphasis is one used as a mantra by many cognitive behavioural therapists that: *'you have to act better before you feel better'*. It is also noteworthy that exercise as a behaviour in its own right now has an evidence base supporting its adoption as a treatment for depression (National Institute for Health and Clinical Excellence, 2004a), although the mechanism of effect is not certain.

Application to new disorders

Together with the integration of the cognitive and the behavioural approaches, and the increasing evidence base, the other main development that has occurred since the 1970s has been the application of cognitive behavioural therapy to more and more problem areas. Beck has continued to spearhead this development with his work in the areas of anxiety disorders (Beck *et al*, 1985), couples therapy (Beck, 1988) and personality disorders (Beck *et al*, 1990). CBT for psychosis has also been a huge growth area as evidenced again by the clear recommendation of the approach in guidelines for the treatment of schizophrenia in the UK (National Institute for Health and Clinical Excellence, 2002).

Other therapies have adopted many of the main elements of CBT. Notable among these have been dialectical behavioural therapy (Linehan *et al*, 1993) and schema therapy (Young *et al*, 2003), which have both been used to treat borderline personality disorder.

Closer links with cognitive psychology

Beck's model of depression was based on clinical observation rather than research evidence. Subsequent years have seen attempts to empirically investigate the underpinnings of his theory. We now know that cognitive behavioural therapy can effectively treat a number of disorders, but we still do not know for sure what the therapy is doing to effect change. These investigations have required much closer dialogue between clinicians and academic cognitive psychologists (Blackburn and Twaddle, 1996).

Researchers have continued to explore the ways in which cognitions become distorted in psychological illness and how these distorted cognitions then act to predispose people to, or maintain, states of mental ill-health. One area of ongoing work has centred on how information can be processed in biased ways – whether that information is from our environment around us, or internally from our thoughts and our memories. Mathews (1997) describes these *information processing biases* within three categories:

1 *selective encoding*: this means that people can have a bias in their selection of information that is congruent upon their mood or emotional state. This can be seen in clients with panic disorder who scan their bodies for sensations that they believe may be evidence of physical threat. They may not register the other sensations information that indicates that there is no threat (Ehlers and Breuer, 1992)
2 *biases in interpretation of meaning*: Mathews (1997) describes how when faced with ambiguous information, people often interpret it in a biased way that fits with their emotional state. Therefore, the panic patient not only selectively attends to the increased heart rate with exercise but also interprets the heart rate as possible evidence of a forthcoming heart attack
3 *memory biases*: not only will the biased conclusions based on selective encoding and meaning interpretation mean that the information passed into memory may be biased in the first place, but Mathews (1997) goes on to describe how even with 'equivalent' memories to draw on, some people preferentially select those memories that correspond with their current emotional state. Depressed patients are biased towards thinking about those memories with a negative theme (Clark and Teasdale, 1985).

Since the early 1990s, another area of research in cognitive psychology has been led by Teasdale and Barnard. Their *'Interacting Cognitive Subsystems* (ICS)' model (Teasdale and Barnard, 1993) has been influential in encouraging debate about the nature of our thoughts, and how this relates to our understanding of how CBT might work. The ICS model states that we have a number of *'minds-in-place'*. Therefore, if an important cognitive theme is activated – such as how we are 'vulnerable' and 'at risk' – then our whole way of functioning and interpreting information will be influenced by that theme. Had we been thinking about another key theme such as the future as exciting and hopeful then our processing of information would be different. Teasdale and Barnard suggest that we all normally move in and out of different 'minds-in-place' as circumstances change, but that in mood disorders we become 'stuck' in that theme without swapping in and out of different themes. This is important because the main 'active ingredient' in CBT suggested by the ICS model may not be to change one or two discrete thoughts. Rather it may be to encourage alternative overall ways of viewing situations, so that the person is no longer as likely to fall back into stereotyped 'minds-in-place', which act to maintain a disorder such as depression.

Future directions

The following are a few of the directions that the authors believe cognitive behavioural therapy will take in the future:

1   the component parts of the cognitive and behavioural model will continue to be open to scientific scrutiny. In time, more complex theoretical constructs such as schemas will be further delineated and investigated. The relationship with cognitive psychology will continue to drive this endeavour. The relative importance of previously under-studied components of depression and anxiety such as rumination and worry will hopefully become clearer, and may link in more closely with the work of Teasdale and colleagues (Teasdale and Barnard, 1993)
2   some of the newer cognitive behavioural informed therapies such as schema therapy (Young *et al*, 2003) and mindfulness-based therapies will continue to develop and find applications in a wider variety of disorders
3   the drive to assess the efficacy of therapy will continue. However, the need to show that therapies work outside of the main academic centres in 'real life' clinical settings will also drive 'effectiveness' research
4   once it can be shown that a therapy is effective then it needs to be broken down to see whether some or all of the component parts of that therapy are required. A good example of a debate surrounding component parts relates to eye movement desensitisation and reprocessing (EMDR) (Shapiro, 1995, *see* Chapter 12). This technique, used in the treatment of PTSD, requires patients to imagine the trauma that they endured, while experiencing lateralised stimuli. It is not yet certain whether the latter are essential or whether the attempt to keep the memory of the trauma in mind (imaginal exposure) is the 'active ingredient'
5   the relationship between psychological treatments, biological treatments such as medication, and biological changes in the central nervous system will become clearer. Already clear changes in the structure and the functioning of

the brain have been observed when applying psychological therapies (Hughes and Riordan, 2006)

6 links will be made with other models, resulting in an enrichment of both theory and practice. For example the relevance of attachment theory to cognitive psychology and cognitive behavioural therapy has recently begun to be explored (Riskind *et al*, 2004)

7 another continued drive is likely to be the attempt to apply cognitive behavioural approaches in more varied formats. This will include the further development of CBT-based group approaches, as well as self-help approaches (Williams and Whitfield, 2001). The latter includes computerised CBT.

MAIN POINTS

- Classic conditioning results in a conditioned response following conditioned stimuli.
- Operant conditioning describes how the consequences of a behaviour lead to an increase or decrease in that behaviour.
- In operant conditioning, the behaviour increases (reinforced) by either reward (positive reinforcement) or the removal of an unpleasant stimulus (negative reinforcement).
- In operant conditioning, the behaviour is reduced by taking away a positive stimulus (frustrative non-reward), or adding a negative stimulus (punishment).
- Social learning was later put forward as an influence, while Beck's cognitive theory of depression further emphasised the influence of thoughts in depression.
- Beck stated that negative cognitions were not only a symptom of depression, but also acted to maintain the depressed state.
- Behavioural approaches have continued to develop, such as the introduction of rewards in the form of activity scheduling in depression.
- Information-processing biases include the selective encoding of information, biases in interpreting the meaning of information and biases of memory.
- The interactive cognitive subsystems (ICS) model states that we have a number of 'minds-in-place' – one is preferentially activated in depression.
- Future directions for CBT will probably include a clarification of the active components of therapy and 'real-life' research in smaller clinical settings outside of academic centres (effectiveness rather than efficacy research).

Further reading

- Beck AT, Rush AJ, Shaw BF and Emery G (1979) *Cognitive Therapy of Depression*. New York: Guilford Press.
- Glassman WE and Hadad M (2004) The behaviourist approach. In: *Approaches to Psychology* (4e). Maidenhead: Open University Press, McGraw-Hill Education, pp. 100–148.

- Hawton K, Salkovskis PM, Kirk J and Clark D (1989) The development and principles of cognitive behavioural treatments. In: Hawton K, Salkovskis PM, Kirk J and Clark D (eds) *Cognitive Behaviour Therapy for Psychiatric Problems: a practical guide*. Oxford: Oxford University Press, pp. 1–12.
- Mathews A (1997) Information-processing biases in emotional disorders. In: Clark DM and Fairburn CG (eds) *Science and Practice of Cognitive Behaviour Therapy*. Oxford: Oxford University Press, pp. 47–66.

Chapter 3

The cognitive behavioural approach in general psychiatry

Introduction • Definition of 'a model' • The formulation in psychiatry • Does this differ from a cognitive behavioural formulation? • Choosing which model to use • The place of the cognitive behavioural model in general psychiatry • Formats of cognitive behavioural interventions • Uses of cognitive behavioural knowledge for the general psychiatrist

Introduction

This chapter aims to examine the ways that cognitive behavioural therapy can have an influence upon general psychiatric practice. By extension it aims to encourage the reader to consider how the principles presented in this book could be integrated within their own understanding and practice of psychiatry.

Definition of 'a model'

The term 'model' is a frequently used term, but what does it actually mean? It is important to understand its meaning in order to be able to understand the context of the 'cognitive behavioural model' within mental health practice. A 'model' is a 'theoretical description of the way a system or process works' (*Collins English Dictionary*, 2003, p. 490). A basic characteristic of a model is that it does not attempt to describe every characteristic of an object or a process – but *only enough to assist in our understanding of some aspect of it*. If we had to describe every aspect of it then we might lose the underlying pattern or process; this is because the model's aim is to present only part of the extremely complex overall picture into an understandable representation. If a model simply described everything that was present it would no longer be a model. An example of a model may be the symbolic representation of a country on a two-dimensional map. This map may display the height of the land, the presence of lakes and rivers and even buildings. But it will not attempt to tell the whole story – if it attempted to it would become overly complex and would no longer be understandable. So the map might display the lie of the land, the buildings or the main features, but will not attempt to show the colours of the fields, the quality of the products made in the factories, the food served in the city centre cafes etc, etc. It can never represent all the characteristics and factors that make up that country. So it is then with mental illness – there will be so many influences, but models are used to map out symbolically only some of the major influences and how they act. This is important when we consider the place of the cognitive behavioural model in our psychiatric practice. There is an example in Box 3.1.

Box 3.1 Case study

Edward grew up in a family of four children in a reasonably wealthy area of a large city. One of his grandparents has a history of schizophrenia, and another has a history of bipolar disorder whose episodes of illness he witnessed throughout his childhood. Three years ago, aged 18 years, Edward started to smoke 'skunk' (a form of cannabis) with friends. He noticed quite early on that the skunk made him suspicious of the actions of others, whereas it did not seem to have such a pronounced effect on his friends. He became psychotic over time, and was seen by the local psychiatric services and prescribed medication that appeared to reduce the psychotic symptoms. Edward decided that he would have to stop meeting with his friends, as he knew they would tempt him subtly into using cannabis again. His activity decreased, he was isolated and he became depressed. His family began to pressurise Edward to go out more and Edward became more and more distressed by the resulting arguments. His symptoms of hearing voices began to get worse and he was eventually admitted to a hostel for the mentally ill where his lifestyle was impoverished. He remained depressed for over two years. He could not afford the luxuries that his 'well' brothers and sisters now afforded themselves in their own newly constituted families in the suburbs.

This not uncommon scenario can be understood from a number of perspectives. That is, we can use a number of different models to explain Edward's illness, and the effect of the illness on his life. Indeed, we can use all of the following (and many more):

- *the disease model*: 'The disease model classifies disorder on the basis of symptom clusters which assume underlying anatomical and physiological change, and imply that there is a unitary disease process corresponding to the symptoms' (Hughes, 1999, p. 24). Using this model we may conclude that Edward has schizophrenia or drug-induced psychosis and that it has a strong genetic (a biological vulnerability to develop psychotic symptoms) and perhaps also an illicit drug causation
- *social models*: social models or social psychology models may emphasise the influence of social groups in determining the conforming behaviour of the individual, such as feeling pressurised to take cannabis, and the resulting isolation when the individual can no longer conform to the 'norms' of the group
- *systemic or family models*: these may attempt to explain the influence of the members of the family unit on the progression of Edward's illness. Concepts such as the power balance within subgroups of the family and reasons for the expressed emotion directed towards Edward may be addressed

- *political models*: these may offer light on the care of the mentally ill within society and the lack of financial support given to carers to maintain care in the family environment rather than resorting to institutionalisation. It may also offer a perspective upon the effects of policing techniques and laws relating to cannabis use
- *cognitive behavioural models*: these may describe among many other things the negative effects of the reduction in activity levels on the maintenance of the depression and the effectiveness of current coping strategies used by Edward in coping with his auditory hallucinations
- *psychodynamic models*: these may relate to Edward's relationship with his family as he was growing up, his view of himself, and his unconscious defence mechanisms that contribute to his current unhappiness.

Various viewpoints or models may be able to explain with validity a part of a given situation. The one we choose to use depends on the view or 'lens' through which we look. Therefore, Edward's situation may be addressed by various means depending on our viewpoint. We could:

- offer him medication if we prioritise the disease model
- lobby for greater controls of cannabis and facilities for the mentally ill by political means
- see the family and look for family dynamics and heightened expressed emotion using systemic models
- provide CBT to teach new coping strategies for hallucinations in accordance with cognitive behavioural models of psychosis
- assess Edward for his suitability for psychodynamic psychotherapy.

All of these may be effective in alleviating Edward's situation, and some may have a place in the management of Edward's 'psychosis'. It is for this reason that the disease model is not encouraged in isolation in psychiatry, and why trainee psychiatrists in many countries such as the UK require exposure to other models and practice such as the various psychological therapies (Whitfield *et al*, 2006). The important point is that there are many ways to minimise the impact of the client's symptoms – providing medication may have a beneficial effect, but then so might stopping access to cannabis and carrying out family work. How then do we choose which model to use to conceptualise our patient's problems?

The formulation in psychiatry

The psychiatric formulation should try and take into account the main models known to have an impact on the presentation of mental health problems. The way that it structures such a diverse mass of factors is by categorising them into the following:

- predisposing factors
- precipitating factors
- maintaining factors.

In essence, this categorisation allows us to consider other angles that are not addressed by only using the disease model. Other factors are considered. It may be that as psychiatrists we cannot address these other factors directly ourselves in treatment, but we might refer to other professionals who can. A formulation that incorporates other models therefore allows us to case manage the patient in a more effective way.

Therefore, Edward's 'psychiatric' formulation would probably include:

- *predisposing factors*:
  - genetic loading
  - his early life experiences including witnessing mental illness in others
- *precipitating factors*:
  - his use of a powerful cannabinoid drug
  - other environmental stressors that occurred at the time of the breakdown, e.g. the high 'expressed emotion' family environment
  - his rejection by his peer group because of the early psychotic symptoms
- *maintaining factors*:
  - low activity levels
  - his isolation from his family (physical separation)
  - his low view of his self-worth relative to others
  - the lack of a peer group, and physical distance from his old peer group
  - his poor compliance with medication.

Some psychiatrists also use the additional structure of 'physical', 'psychological' and 'social' factors in addition to the above 'predisposing', 'precipitating', and 'maintaining' factor structure. Combining the two gives us Table 3.1, which shows causal factors for Edward.

Table 3.1 Edward's 'psychiatric formulation'

	Physical	*Psychological*	*Social*
Predisposing factors	Genetic loading	Witnessing mental illness in his childhood	The free availability of cannabinoids in his peer group
Precipitating factors	His use of the cannabinoid drug	1 The high expressed emotion in the family 2 The effect of rejection by his peer group	The effects of stigma concerning mental health symptoms
Maintaining factors	Poor compliance with medication	1 Low activity levels 2 His view of self compared with others	1 Physical isolation from his peer group 2 Distance from his family 3 His lack of financial resources

Does this differ from a cognitive behavioural formulation?

Writing a general psychiatric formulation as described above does differ from the cognitive behavioural formulations that can be requested for example in membership examinations. The formation of a cognitive behavioural formulation is described in Chapter 5. It relies upon the use of information that is directly relevant to the cognitive behavioural understanding of the illness in question. So, a cognitive behavioural formulation of a man with depression for example would discuss cognitive distortions/errors typical of the depressed state, and behaviours that were acting to maintain the low mood. Keeping to the cognitive behavioural model does, however, mean that we will choose to omit some of the information that is not contained within the cognitive behavioural model!

Choosing which model to use

Although in psychiatry the general formulation may include physical (including genetic and medication), psychological and social factors, when it comes to devising a specific psychological therapy intervention there are advantages to working to a specialist formulation based on only one model. There is little sense in devising a mixed psychodynamic and cognitive behavioural formulation, for example. Constructing a 'pure' formulation based on only one model is recommended for the following reasons:

- to allow the formulation to be constructed in accordance with the relevant model. This is important if the validity of the model in a given form has been experimentally validated
- the approaches of the different models of treatment may conflict for any given problem. It therefore makes sense to tailor the formulation to one treatment model only
- eclecticism in psychotherapy is a controversial subject. It is probably the case that patients understand the approach best if only one model is used and if that model is explained to the patient in a clear and structured formulation.

If then you decide to undertake psychological therapy for your patient, which therapy model do you choose? The following are some factors that will help you choose – there are actually many more influences that are debated between psychotherapists but which are outside the remit of this book:

- the *evidence base for the general illness area* that the client presents with. For example, there is good evidence to support CBT as the primary treatment for panic disorder (National Institute for Health and Clinical Excellence, 2004b), but a complex presentation with personality problems may be best formulated and treated using either a CBT-based approach or psychodynamic psychotherapy
- the *predominant causal factors* may fit best within the remit of one model over the others. For example, a couple who are having relationship problems and who present with significant symptoms of depression may be best understood using a systemic model and may therefore be best treated using a family or couples therapy. This would also fit with the evidence base in that couples therapy is

mentioned as an evidence-based treatment for depression in the NICE guidelines (National Institute for Health and Clinical Excellence, 2004a)

- patients and their families often have a view on the model of psychological therapy with which they would like to work. *Choice* is now an important part of the delivery of services within the health sector. Some will have had one form of therapy and worked well with it in the past. Others may have failed with a form of therapy and wish to try a different approach
- if a specific therapist is being asked to deliver the therapy then obviously their ability to work within different models will be constrained by the *training that they have received*. It may also be constrained by the accreditation that they have with *professional bodies* which monitor psychotherapy practice, e.g. BABCP for cognitive behavioural psychotherapists
- finally, in many areas only some *models of therapy will be available*. This is particularly the case in more rural regions. For example, until recently there were no private BABCP-accredited psychotherapists listed by the BABCP website covering a huge area of Southern Scotland (Dumfries and Galloway and Borders). In comparison at the time of writing this book there are 74 such private therapists serving Greater London! Therapist provision within the NHS in the UK is similarly quite patchy (as we understand it is in most countries).

The place of the cognitive behavioural model in general psychiatry

If choosing a model of therapy, constructing a formulation in accordance with that model, and then delivering that specific therapy is recommended, then where does this leave the general psychiatrist who may not have the time or the training to provide specialist psychotherapy? This is a commonly debated question (Whitfield *et al*, 2006). A cognitive behavioural understanding of the causation and maintenance of mental illness is still judged important even among those psychiatrists trained in CBT who are not able to carry out formal therapy (Ashworth *et al*, 1999). CBT-informed psychiatric practice is valued. To answer why this might be we need to look at the ways in which CBT is delivered in mental health practice.

Formats of cognitive behavioural interventions

Cognitive behavioural therapy has flourished, no doubt in part due to the evidence base that supports its use. The number of people accredited in the practice of cognitive and behavioural psychotherapies in the UK has been steadily rising towards the 1000 mark (see the British Association for Behavioural and Cognitive Psychotherapies (BABCP) at babcp.org.uk). To a purist, CBT can only be delivered by one therapist to one client in the traditional manner. More recently this view has been challenged, as the demand for therapy outstrips the capacity for the available therapists to meet it (Williams and Whitfield, 2001). Cognitive behavioural treatments are therefore increasing in range, and include the following:

- *group cognitive behavioural therapy*: the effectiveness of this mode of providing a cognitive behavioural understanding to clients has been researched less than for

CBT provided on an individual basis. There may be advantages in providing CBT in this format for some diagnostic areas, such as social phobia. Here the presence of other clients with similar problems allows the whole group to investigate and challenge each other's faulty assumptions in a way that might not be so powerful in individual treatment. Group-based interventions have increasingly been used in the informal sector in the UK (including by charities such as the Manic Depression Fellowship). Some health sector departments also run pre-dominantly group-based CBT service delivery

- *CBT-based self-help*: self-help has increased in popularity in the last decade. Most self-help materials used in the health sector for mental health problems are CBT based (Whitfield and Williams, 2003). There is a significant evidence base now supporting the use of self-help for common mental health problems such as depression and anxiety (Proudfoot *et al*, 2003). Although self-help can be delivered by a wide variety of means including by audiocassette and videotape, it is book-based (bibliotherapy) and computer-based self-help that have recently attracted the most attention. Computerised CBT (CCBT) programmes such as *Beating the Blues* (www.ultrasis.com/pdf/btb_overview.pdf) and *Overcoming Depression* are widely marketed. Most of the materials from *Overcoming Depression* are available on the Internet at: www.livinglifetothefull.co.uk. At the present time, however, given the added costs of providing and maintaining computerised provision of CBT, some services choose written self-help instead

- *CBT-informed specific interventions*: increasingly it has been acknowledged that patients may benefit from engaging in a cognitive behavioural intervention without needing to undergo a full course of cognitive behavioural therapy. Some community mental health teams (CMHTs) have been trained in the delivery of simple CBT-based interventions using written self-help materials to guide them. In Glasgow there have been a number of training courses such as the SPIRIT (Structured Psychosocial InteRventions In Teams) project in secondary care and the START project (Self-help Training Access Resource Team) in primary care, training staff in self-help-based CBT interventions (Chris Williams, University of Glasgow, personal communication). Such interventions may include assisting patients to reduce their use of avoidance as a coping strategy or identifying and challenging extreme and unhelpful thinking (Williams and Garland, 2002). Sometimes CMHT staff can also undertake cognitive behavioural interventions such as increasing activity levels under the supervision of a CBT-trained staff member who may be a psychiatrist. Often this is most useful when it supplements or continues the work of formal cognitive behavioural therapy undertaken elsewhere.

The above CBT interventions can be viewed along a spectrum of complexity, with CBT-based self-help at one end through to longer-term specialist cognitive behavioural therapy at the other. These different levels of complexity of intervention can be operated within a '*stepped care*' model of service delivery where more simple and less intrusive interventions are offered first, before offering more complex interventions only if the earlier interventions are not effective. Self-help is more commonly offered as an initial intervention, with group or individual CBT only offered as a later step if necessary. Although the concept of stepped care is an attractive one, its place within mental health provision has still to be proven (Bower and Gilbody, 2005).

Different levels or complexity of CBT delivery correspond with *differing levels of training requirements*. These range from the postgraduate diploma or masters' level most commonly required for the specialist cognitive therapist, through to the 35–40 hours of training equipping staff to deliver basic CBT-based self-help materials, as occurs with the SPIRIT project in Glasgow.

Uses of cognitive behavioural knowledge for the general psychiatrist

Finally, we can reconsider why the general psychiatrist would benefit from cognitive behavioural training. Here are some of the ways in which it might be used:

- to be able to look at a situation through a new 'lens' can help the psychiatrist understand complex problems from a different angle
- to understand the role and place of cognitive behavioural interventions within the overall management strategy for the patient. Knowing who to refer and when to refer is an important part of this, and comes from personal experience with the approach
- psychiatrists with an interest in CBT can supervise other CMHT staff members to carry out cognitive behavioural interventions or supervise more formal cognitive behavioural therapy
- to train junior psychiatrists in the practice of CBT. A recent survey of the 60 or so psychiatrists in Scotland who have been trained to a specialist level in CBT showed that about half were trainers and supervisors of junior doctors and other team members in CBT (Whitfield *et al*, 2006)
- to carry out cognitive behavioural therapy with more complex patients where a knowledge of psychiatry aids management. Patients with severe anorexia or personality disorders are examples where consultant psychiatrists may be best placed to personally undertake the therapy.

MAIN POINTS

- Models are a symbolic representation of a subject and therefore will not include *all* potentially relevant information.
- The cognitive behavioural model looks at a subject from one angle; other models concentrate upon other aspects.
- Models are the structure upon which we devise a formulation for the individual patient.
- In general psychiatry the formulation categorises causal factors into predisposing, precipitating and maintaining factors. These factors can also be further categorised into physical, psychological and social factors.
- Constructing a formulation based upon the underlying theoretical model is necessary in psychotherapy.

- The choice of which model of psychological therapy to use will depend on the evidence base for that disorder, the predominant apparent causal factors, patient choice, the patient's previous response to therapy, and the local availability of therapists with the necessary training and accreditation.
- CBT can be delivered in different formats including in groups, using self-help materials (including computerised CBT), and by training staff in specific cognitive behavioural interventions.
- The benefits of a cognitive behavioural training for the general psychiatrist include a knowledge of who to refer for cognitive behavioural therapy, and an ability to train and to supervise other team members in this approach.

Further reading

- Bower P and Gilbody S (2005) Stepped care in psychological therapies: access, effectiveness and efficiency. Narrative literature review. *British Journal of Psychiatry* 186: 11–17.
- Royal College of Psychiatrists (2002) Requirements for psychotherapy training as part of basic specialist training. www.rcpsych.ac.uk/PDF/ptBasic.pdf.
- Whitfield G, Connolly M, Davidson A and Williams C (2006) Use of cognitive-behavioural therapy skills among trained psychiatrists. *Psychiatric Bulletin* 30: 58–61.

Chapter 4

Evidence base for cognitive behavioural therapy

> Introduction • Depression • Anxiety disorders • Obsessive-compulsive
> disorder • Post-traumatic stress disorder • Schizophrenia and related
> psychoses • Eating disorders • Bipolar disorder • Borderline personality
> disorder

Introduction

This chapter provides a brief overview of the current evidence base for cognitive
behavioural therapy as applied to each of the major disorder areas outlined later in
the book. The review is not a formal systematic review in that we have not
presented all potential papers relevant to the diagnostic areas. Rather we have
attempted to present the major points and provide key references where more
detailed information can be accessed. In addition, the most up-to-date guidelines
from the National Institute of Health and Clinical Excellence (NICE), at least those
that apply to CBT, are also outlined. These are likely to exert increasing influence
on treatment provision in the future – certainly within the UK. Because the NICE
guidelines are constantly evolving, the authors recommend that the reader checks
the current guidelines at nice.org.uk, as the information outlined in this chapter
may become superseded with subsequent versions of the published NICE guidelines. After the major NICE recommendation points have been outlined, we
include *ratings for the strength of supporting evidence* that NICE provide for each
recommendation point. For example, in the NICE guidelines on depression
(2004a) there is a recommendation point that treatment-resistant depression
should be treated with a combination of medication and CBT. The evidence that
supports this recommendation point is at a 'B' level rating. The NICE guidelines
draw on a number of different quality 'levels'. These in turn draw on different
categories of evidence. Both the levels of strength of evidence and the categories of
evidence on which they are based are described in Box 4.1.

> **Box 4.1   The NICE evidence classification and rating system**
>
> **Category of evidence**
>
> - *Ia*: from meta-analyses of randomised controlled trials (RCTs)
> - *Ib*: from at least one RCT

- *IIa*: from at least one controlled study without randomisation
- *IIb*: from at least one other type of quasi-experimental study
- *III*: from descriptive studies (e.g. comparative, correlation and case-control studies)
- *IV*: from expert committee reports or opinions, or clinical experience of respected authority or both

Ratings for strength of supporting evidence

- *A*: directly based on Category I evidence
- *B*: directly based on Category II evidence or extrapolated from Category I evidence
- *C*: directly based on Category III evidence or extrapolated from Category II evidence
- *D*: directly based on Category IV evidence or extrapolated from Category III evidence

GPP: in addition, some of the guidelines have included a *'GPP'* strength of supporting evidence. This stands for 'good practice points'. It means that the recommendation is based on the clinical experience of the *Guideline Development Group (GDG)* – that is the group of interested professionals who meet to consider the evidence and who thus collate the guidelines.

The majority of outcome data supporting the use of CBT is termed *'efficacy'* data rather than *'effectiveness'* data. The former refers to evidence from trials carried out mainly in specialist academic settings. The latter refers to data from 'routine settings' that are more representative of the treatments that most patients receive worldwide. In reality many studies have some characteristics of 'efficacy' design and others of 'effectiveness' design (Chambless and Peterman, 2004). A major challenge for all researchers in psychotherapy is to increase the proportion of studies that have been completed in circumstances that more accurately reflect the way that treatment is routinely delivered.

Depression

A few trials investigating the treatment of depression have been particularly influential (Roth and Fonagy, 2005). The best known of these is probably the *National Institute of Mental Health (NIMH) study* (Elkin, 1994), which used a relatively large US study population (239 entrants) randomised to four arms of treatment: CBT, IPT, imipramine plus 'clinical management' and placebo plus 'clinical management'. Clinical management comprised weekly meetings of 20–30 minutes in addition to further support and advice when requested. This went some way to equalise the amount of face-to-face contact between the four treatments so that the specific effects of the therapies could be tested. Patients in all four groups improved, but there were no significant differences in outcome between the groups (although controversy surrounds the results). Surprisingly few of the recovered patients from all groups remained well at 18 months' follow-up (Shea *et al*, 1992). This has led to the conclusion that 16 weeks of treatment was not long enough for this population, over half of whom had been depressed for over 6 months (Roth and Fonagy, 2005).

Encouraging outcomes for the psychological treatment of depression were shown by another landmark US-based trial, which indicated that 20 sessions of CBT could be as effective as imipramine (Evans *et al*, 1992). Combining CBT and antidepressant treatments did not result in significantly improved outcomes. The relapse rate at follow-up two years later was only 18% in the CBT group, almost half that in the imipramine-treated group who continued imipramine after treatment (at 32%) and much lower than those who had been given imipramine but who discontinued it at the end of the treatment phase (50% relapse rate). This trial pointed to trends that have been repeated by more recent studies, in particular the long-term benefits seen with CBT.

In the UK the so-called '*Sheffield Psychotherapy Project*' has been similarly influential (Shapiro *et al*, 1994). One hundred and seventeen patients completed treatment with either CBT or a form of therapy called '*psychodynamic-interpersonal therapy*' (PI). Once again, the results surprised many in that there was no overall significant difference between the outcomes of the two groups of treated patients at the end of treatment. However, the patients who had only eight sessions of PI did not do so well at 12 months' follow-up, compared to those who had had 16 sessions of PI, or for that matter those who had had either 8 or 16 sessions of CBT (Shapiro *et al*, 1995). Those who initially presented with severe depression required longer treatments (16 rather than 8 sessions) and were more at risk of relapse.

A *meta-analysis* looking at short-term psychological treatments for depression found equivalent outcomes for CBT and IPT, but CBT appeared to give superior outcomes relative to both psychodynamic therapy and supportive therapy (Churchill *et al*, 2001). Meanwhile, a review of *group treatments for depression* (mainly based on CBT approaches) found no significant difference in outcome between therapy delivered on an individual and on a group basis (McDermut *et al*, 2001). Another delivery method for CBT-type interventions has been via *computerised CBT* (CCBT) and *written self-help (bibliotherapy)*. Although some work has shown that the outcomes of patients using written self-help can be equivalent to those who have individual CBT with a therapist (e.g. Cuijpers, 1997), the majority of the available written self-help materials have not been assessed. Few large trials have been carried out for *CCBT*. One noteworthy trial showed improved outcomes with the use of a computer programme compared to treatment as usual, benefits that continued at 6 months' follow-up (Proudfoot *et al*, 2003).

As Evans *et al* (1992) indicated, CBT has the potential to *reduce the relapse rates* of patients with depression (probably because it teaches techniques to protect against further episodes). The NIMH study did not show superior longer-term outcomes with CBT over other treatments (Shea *et al*, 1992); however, another more recent trial on participants who had previously recovered from depression (Paykel *et al*, 1999; Paykel, 2001) showed reduced rates of subsequent relapse in those patients who had been treated with CBT. The pattern whereby patients who have responded to CBT relapse on follow-up significantly less often than patients who have responded to medication but stopped taking it has been shown by Hollon *et al* (2005). This study was all the more important in that it had sizable study populations who also had *moderate-to-severe depression*. They found that the relapse rate of patients continued on medication was equivalent to that of those who had finished CBT (slightly better outcomes for medication than the trial by Evans *et al* (1992). However, this raises questions about the *longer-term cost-effectiveness of medication* when it appears to require ongoing prescribing to protect against further episodes (unlike CBT which seems to protect after a one-off series of sessions; Hollon and DeRubeis, 2004). Whether medication or psychological therapy is the cheaper option is controversial (*see* Pirraglia *et al*, 2004 for a systematic review).

Another more recent development has been '*mindfulness-based cognitive therapy*', which also aims to reduce relapse rates in depression (Teasdale, 1999). Outcome studies are still few in number, but a trial in which patients who had suffered two or more episodes of depression were given this therapy showed a reduced relapse rate (over 60 weeks) compared to treatment as usual (Teasdale *et al*, 2000). Those who were *younger* when they first became depressed, and those who had suffered a *greater number of relapses* benefited the most.

A large trial (650 participants) has also shown significant benefit from a form of CBT-based therapy as a treatment of *chronic depression* (Keller *et al*, 2000). This trial found that those who had both an antidepressant medication and psychological therapy did better than those who had received only one or the other. However, for depression in general, the issue of whether a *combination of CBT and medication* results in outcomes that are superior to either treatment alone is controversial (Roth and Fonagy, 2005). Others have not observed benefits from combining medication with talking treatments (e.g. Evans *et al*, 1992, *see* above), although the evidence for combination treatments is stronger for more severe depression (Thase *et al*, 1997).

Moderate-to-severe depression in general has been the subject of work by DeRubeis and colleagues (DeRubeis *et al*, 1999, 2005; Hollon *et al*, 2005). Previously it had been considered that severe depression should be preferentially treated with medication (American Psychiatric Association, 2000). DeRubeis *et al* (2005) showed that response rates at 8 weeks after either CBT treatment or treatment with medication were equivalent and superior to placebo. At 16 weeks, the equivalency continued (at most trial centres), suggesting that CBT can be an effective treatment for this more severe group. It is acknowledged, however, that in moderate-to-severe depression, there is currently more of an evidence base supporting treatment with antidepressant medication than with CBT. In terms of *inpatient care*, one trial showed that the addition of 12 sessions of group CBT to the normal hospital management of depression (including medication), results in significantly reduced rates of depression on discharge (Bowers, 1990).

CBT can be effective with *different age groups*. Child and adolescent outcomes are not addressed in this book, but there is evidence that CBT can be effective for mild to moderate depression in *old age* (Thompson *et al*, 2001). There is less evidence that CBT is effective in *dysthymic disorder* at any age, but this is an area of interest as many of these patients go on to develop a full-blown depressive episode, so-called '*double depression*' (Wells *et al*, 1992).

In terms of other treatments for depression, *couple therapies* (which may be CBT based) may be more efficacious than individual therapies when relationship issues are particularly relevant to the patient's mood disorder (e.g. Emanuels-Zuurveen and Emmelkamp, 1996). There is also evidence for *problem-solving approaches* (Mynors-Wallis *et al*, 2000) and *non-directive counselling* (e.g. Ward *et al*, 2000) in *mild-to-moderate depression in primary care*.

NICE Guidelines CG023: depression (NICE 2004a)

These guidelines provide recommendations on the treatment of depression in primary and secondary care within a *stepped care model*. By 'stepped care' it presupposes that patients usually present at a low step, perhaps in a routine general practitioner (GP) surgery appointment, but will potentially 'move up' the steps receiving treatment from higher steps as required. It separates depression into mild, moderate-to-severe, treatment-resistant, recurrent and chronic.

Mild depression

- A major element of the management of mild depression is *'watchful waiting'*, whereby patients are given an appointment two weeks after presenting to assess whether the mild symptoms have subsided. Management includes the provision of information about *exercise* (C), *sleep hygiene* (C) and *anxiety management* (C).
- Clients with mild depression may be treated using *CBT-based guided self-help* (B). The self-help is written (bibliotherapy), and the 'guided' refers to the access to a healthcare worker who introduces the materials and is on-hand to review progress. The self-help should progress over 6 to 9 weeks.

Short-term psychological treatment in both mild and moderate depression

- The recommended psychological approach is the use of *6 to 8 sessions* over 10 to 12 weeks of therapies with a *specific focus on the depression*, such as brief CBT, counselling and problem-solving therapy (B). Which model is chosen will depend on a number of factors such as personal preference. The guidelines elaborate that staff providing the therapy need to be *competent and experienced* (GPP), and need to develop and maintain a *therapeutic alliance* in order to achieve good outcomes (C).

Moderate-to-severe depression

- To use the wording of the guidelines:

  'When considering individual psychological treatments for moderate, severe and treatment-resistant depression, the treatment of choice is CBT. IPT should be considered if the patient expresses a preference for it or if, in the view of the healthcare professional, the patient may benefit from it' (B) (NICE 2004a, p. 27, point 1.5.3.1).

- The recommended duration of therapy is longer than for milder depression, (i.e. usually *16–20 sessions*) over 6 to 9 months (B). The principles already outlined in terms of the choice of therapy, competence and experience of the staff and the therapeutic alliance still apply.
- The guidelines state that those with moderate or severe depression should be offered CBT when, for whatever reason, they do not take antidepressant medication (B). Similarly, CBT may be offered to those who have not had a very good response to other treatments such as antidepressants in the past (C).
- They recommend twice-weekly therapy in the first month for severely depressed patients, and clear follow-up, typically 2–4 sessions over a year, in patients who have responded to CBT (C).

- *A combination of antidepressants and individual CBT should be used when patients initially present with severe depression*. The combination is more cost-effective than either treatment on its own (B).

Treatment-resistant depression

- For the group of patients who relapse while still taking or after ending anti-depressant medication, the guidelines suggest the combination of CBT with continued antidepressant medication (B).

Recurrent depression

- Similarly, CBT is recommended for patients who recurrently relapse despite antidepressant medication, or who wish to have psychological therapy instead of medication (C).
- Likewise if a patient has a previous history of relapse but also has a poor or limited response to other treatments then they should also be considered for CBT (B).
- If the patient is similarly prone to relapse with moderate-to-severe depression, but cannot or does not wish to continue a treatment that has been successful, then they should be considered for 'maintenance CBT' (B).
- Finally, the guidelines note that a form of CBT (*mindfulness-based CBT*), which is usually delivered in groups, may be considered for people who are currently well but have previously suffered three or more episodes of depression. This may significantly reduce the likelihood of future relapse (B).

Chronic depression

- This is where the diagnosable depression has been present for at least 2 years. The recommendation is for combined treatment with antidepressant medication and CBT (A).

Other psychological interventions

- The guidelines recommend consideration of *couple-focused therapy* when the depressed patient has a regular partner and when they have also not benefited from a brief intervention given on an individual basis (B).
- Where depression is complicated by 'complex co-morbidities' it may be appropriate to use *psychodynamic psychotherapy* (C).
- Befriending by providing social support should be considered as an option in addition to medication and CBT in chronic depression (C).

NICE Review of Technology Appraisal 97: Computerised Cognitive Behaviour Therapy for Depression and Anxiety (NICE, 2006a)

This appraisal looked at the use of five specific computer packages – one for panic/phobias called 'FearFighter', one for OCD called 'OCFighter', and three for depression ('COPE', 'Overcoming Depression' and 'Beating the Blues'). The recommendations are to be read and interpreted in conjunction with the NICE guidelines on depression (NICE, 2004a), anxiety (NICE, 2004b) and OCD (NICE, 2005a).

The guidelines recommend 'Beating the Blues' for the management of mild and moderate depression, but state that at present there is insufficient evidence to recommend 'COPE' and 'Overcoming Depression' except as part of effectiveness trials.

'Fearfighter' is recommended for phobia and panic, but OCFighter is not recommended as an option in the management of OCD (however people already using it should have the option of continuing to do so until it is judged by professionals to be appropriate to stop).

Anxiety disorders

Simple phobias

The techniques with the most evidence supporting their use in the treatment of *simple phobias* are all *exposure-based* (Antony and Barlow, 2001). Roth and Fonagy (2005) estimate that 70–85% of patients with simple phobias show clinically significant benefit with these techniques. Exposure techniques now generally refer to graded exposure *in vivo* to the feared object. This can be real or imagined exposure. Virtual reality is also now used as a form of exposure – particularly for flying phobias. *Exposure techniques* are classed as *behaviour therapy* – cognitive techniques are less frequently used for simple phobias. The therapist can supervise the exposure (therapist-directed exposure), or the patients can carry out the exposure themselves without supervision (self-directed exposure). Generally better outcomes are achieved with *therapist-directed exposure* (Öst *et al*, 1991). There is also evidence that a few longer-exposure sessions (often over an hour) can be as effective as shorter, more frequent sessions (Öst, 1989). *Benzodiazepine* use may be effective in the shorter term, but the benefits reduce over time so that longer-term behaviour therapy (which includes exposure) is more effective over the long term (Thom *et al*, 2000). In fact, there is evidence that using benzodiazepines for simple phobias concurrently with behaviour therapy lowers the effectiveness of the behaviour therapy (Wilhelm and Roth, 1997). This is probably because they 'numb' the individual and impair their ability to habituate to the associated anxiety. For this reason, many centres require patients to be *weaned off benzodiazepines* before starting exposure work.

Social phobia

There is clear evidence supporting the use of both psychotropic medications and varying forms of CBT (*see* Rodebaugh *et al*, 2004 for review). Comparison studies between different medications and different psychological approaches are rare, and the longer-term outcomes for treatment with medication are not clear (Fedoroff and Taylor, 2001). In one of the few comparisons with non-CBT psychological approaches, CBT was found to be more effective than supportive therapy (Cottraux *et al*, 2000).

Moreno *et al* (2001) completed a meta-analysis comparing the outcomes of exposure alone (behavioural technique), cognitive restructuring alone (cognitive technique), and social skills training. The results of the three were equivalent, raising unanswered questions about what the active ingredients are in the CBT treatment of social phobia. Moreno and colleagues suggest that the active ingredient that is common in most CBT approaches is the exposure to the feared stimulus of performing in front of others.

There is also uncertainty about the relative effectiveness of individually administered and group-administered CBT for social phobia. Although it may be
hypothesised that groups would be an effective format (to allow exposure to the
feared stimulus) the results have varied (e.g. Heimberg *et al*, 1990; Moreno *et al*,
2001; Stangier *et al*, 2003).

Panic disorder

Of all anxiety disorders, it is for *panic disorder* where there is the most evidence
supporting the use of CBT. Patients with panic seem to *respond well* to CBT
compared to those with some other anxiety disorders such as generalised anxiety
disorder (GAD). In one meta-analysis, 85% of clients with panic disorder
responded to CBT (Chambless and Gillis, 1993). There are now many individual
studies, reviews and meta-analyses addressing panic disorder (both with and
without agoraphobia). It has been concluded that the panic symptoms respond
to the cognitive elements of CBT (primarily teaching the client not to misinterpret
the bodily symptoms of panic), while the agoraphobic avoidance responds to the
behavioural method of exposure (Roth and Fonagy, 2005). Exposing the patient
literally to the feared situations (*'in vivo exposure'*) leads to better outcomes
compared to *'imaginal exposure'*, where the patient simply imagines being in the
feared and avoided situations (Trull *et al*, 1988).

Questions that remain unanswered include the *number of CBT sessions* that are
required, *who should deliver* the CBT and *where it should be delivered*, and the *role of
medication* as an alternative or adjunctive treatment to CBT. Some studies have
shown equivalent results to the traditional 14-session CBT treatments when fewer
face-to-face sessions are delivered (approximately 6–8) in conjunction with
written manuals or hand-held computers (Clark *et al*, 1999; Kenardy *et al*, 2003).
Others have gone further and instructed the use of written self-help materials
(*bibliotherapy*) without offering any one-to-one therapy, although the results have
varied (Lidren *et al*, 1994; Sharp *et al*, 2000). The potential use of computerised self-
help has been shown with the programme 'FearFighter' (see NICE *Technology
Appraisal 97*, NICE 2006a) described earlier in this book, p. 37).

The issue of who should deliver CBT (and where) has centered on the potential
role of *primary care workers*. These have included GPs themselves, who have been
shown to be capable of delivering CBT for panic disorder with equivalent outcomes
to secondary care psychotherapists (van Boeijen *et al*, 2005).

In terms of whether *CBT or medication* should be used for panic disorder, one
observed pattern is that antidepressant medication (e.g. SSRIs and tricyclics)
provides equivalent or even superior benefits relative to CBT, but that CBT-treated
clients maintain these benefits more often than those treated solely with medication (e.g. Barlow *et al*, 2000). The debate about whether *antidepressant medication in
addition to psychotherapy (predominantly CBT)* is better than either alone has been
addressed by Furukawa *et al* (2006) in a meta-analysis. Based on 21 trials they
concluded that in the *acute phase*, combined therapy was superior to either antidepressant medication or psychotherapy alone. After termination of the acute-
phase treatment, the combined therapy was as effective as psychotherapy, but
more effective than pharmacotherapy alone. In other words this again points to the
superior longer-term outcomes of talking treatments for panic disorder compared

to drug treatments, and suggests that combined CBT and drug treatment gives better short-term outcomes but no better outcome that CBT by itself at follow-up. However, it should be noted that this analysis did include a number of models of therapy under the 'psychotherapy' label, which limits the conclusions that can be specifically taken for CBT.

Finally, in common with the treatment of phobias, *benzodiazepines may impair the beneficial effects of exposure-based therapies* in panic disorder (Marks *et al*, 1993).

Generalised anxiety disorder

Although the evidence base for CBT in GAD is not as extensive as it is for panic disorder, a number of both efficacy and effectiveness trials have been concluded over the last decade supporting the use of CBT (*see* Chambless and Peterman (2004) for a meta-analysis). Trials show *clear clinical improvement with CBT*, on a par with medication, but superior to outcomes with psychodynamic therapy and non-directive counselling-type therapy (e.g. Durham *et al*, 1994; Fisher and Durham, 1999; Borkovec and Ruscio, 2001 and Gould *et al*, 1997 for a meta-analysis of CBT versus medication). The *impact of medication* is not clearly described in this area. Chambless and Peterman (2004) point to the fact that many studies that have measured the impact of CBT have allowed patients to concurrently continue on medication. This may have even overestimated the impact of the CBT. Fisher and Durham (1999) found that just over half of the clients treated with either CBT or individual applied relaxation were well 6 months after treatment. The rates of recovery for the other models of therapy were lower still. This lower recovery rate also applied to behaviour therapy – suggesting that the cognitive element of CBT is required for a complex disorder such as GAD. This latter finding was not, however, observed in the meta-analysis of Chambless and Peterman (2004). Roth and Fonagy (2005) conclude that the *best outcomes in GAD are observed with CBT and applied relaxation*. They confirm the findings of Fisher and Durham (1999) that *only 50 to 65% of treated clients show 'clinically significant improvement'*, even after using these treatments, and many of those who do benefit will not do so completely, but will continue to show some features of illness. Chambless and Peterman (2004) comment on these relatively 'sobering' outcomes (at least compared to panic disorder), stating that CBT cannot currently be viewed as a 'panacea' for GAD (p. 111). This meta-analysis also found that *elderly patients with GAD did worse* than their younger counterparts. It is fair to say that GAD requires further research, not only into the outcomes of different treatment strategies but also into the basic way in which the disorder is conceptualised, and the influence of co-morbidities such as panic and depression. GAD has *origins in childhood*, possibly in attachment styles, which influence the development of an *ongoing perception of threat and vulnerability* throughout adult life (Williams and Riskind, 2004). This perception becomes entrenched, and its *chronic nature* may help to explain not only the mediocre outcomes with treatment but also the particularly poor outcomes in the elderly who have suffered with the disorder for longer (Chambless and Peterman, 2004).

NICE guidelines CG022: anxiety (NICE, 2004b)

The guidelines state that there are advantages to treating anxiety disorders in *primary care*. They also state that:

- *psychological therapy, medication* and *self-help* have all been shown to be effective in both GAD and panic disorder (A)
- there is evidence of *longer duration of effect in psychological therapies* compared to medication (A)
- *medication* is similarly observed to have longer-lasting effects than *self-help* (A).

The guidelines do state, however, that some forms of treatment, such as CBT, may not be locally available (or may not be acceptable to the patient) so that treatment decisions may need to be based on a 'pragmatic discussion' between clinician and patient.

CBT for panic

With specific reference to CBT for panic, NICE guidelines recommend that CBT should be used (A).

They do, however, recommend that the CBT should be delivered in specific ways:

- by therapists who are suitably supervised and suitably trained and who can closely adhere to treatment protocols (A)
- it should last for between 7 and 14 hours (A)
- for most people it should be given in weekly sessions lasting 1–2 hours, and overall it should last less than 4 months from beginning to end (B)
- if 'briefer CBT' is used (approximately 7 hours of therapy) then it needs to be:
  - supplemented with appropriate focused information and tasks (A)
  - designed to integrate with structured self-help materials (D)
- more intensive CBT over a very short period may be appropriately used for some patients (C).

CBT for GAD

- In common with panic disorder, there is a clear recommendation that CBT should be used for GAD (A).
- Similarly there are recommendations about the way that the CBT is delivered. These are identical to those described above for panic disorder except that:
  - the therapy should last longer than for the treatment of panic – between 16 and 20 hours (A)
  - briefer CBT is described as being between 8 and 10 sessions. Once again the provisos 'to supplement with appropriate focused information and tasks' (A) and to be 'designed to integrate with structured self-help materials' (D), still apply
  - there is no mention of 'intensive CBT'.

Other CBT delivery methods

- The guidelines state that CBT-based written self-help (bibliotherapy) should be offered for both panic disorder and GAD (A).
- For GAD, the guidelines suggest consideration of large-group CBT (C).

- In addition, information about support groups that may be run on CBT principles should be provided for both GAD and panic disorder (D).

(Note also NICE 2006a Technology Appraisal 97: *Computerised Cognitive Behaviour Therapy for Depression and Anxiety* (p. 37).)

Obsessive-compulsive disorder

Of all the psychological approaches it is the cognitive and behavioural therapies that have been the most researched in the area of obsessive–compulsive disorder (OCD). More specifically, *exposure and response prevention* (ERP) (a behavioural approach) has more evidence supporting its use in this disorder than any other psychological approach. Earlier studies showed that both the exposure and the response-prevention elements were required – neither simply exposing the patient to the stimulus (that precipitates the compulsion), nor simply stopping the client from carrying out their compulsion without prior exposure is effective (e.g. Foa *et al* 1980). Meta-analyses (e.g. Kobak *et al*, 1998) confirm that ERP is an effective treatment for OCD. The results of the efficacy of antidepressant medication compared to ERP have been inconclusive (e.g. Foa *et al*, 2005, reviewed in the NICE guidelines CG031, NICE 2005a). However, the *relapse rate after a course of ERP has been shown to be significantly lower* than the relapse rate observed after stopping clomipramine (Öst, 1989; Pato *et al*, 1988). There is some evidence (five relevant studies were reviewed in the NICE guidelines CG031) that a combination of antidepressant medication and ERP can result in greater improvement than either alone. However, this remains an uncertain area that requires further research (Heyman *et al*, 2006).

It must be remembered that OCD is a difficult disorder to eradicate completely. Although ERP-based CBT has overall response rates of up to 85% (Foa and Goldstein, 1978), these response rates are lower at the severe end of the spectrum. Up to 40% of patients who present to psychiatrists do not adequately respond to either CBT, or medication, or a combination of both (Heyman *et al*, 2006). It has been shown that significant residual symptoms remain at follow-up between 1 and 6 years after treatment has ended (O'Sullivan and Marks, 1991). As might be expected, those who are left inadequately treated, and continue to have *residual symptoms of OCD* subsequently have an increased rate of full relapse (Foa and Kozak, 1996).

A respected review of the literature (Roth and Fonagy, 2005) supports the use of ERP in specific ways:

- it should incorporate the use of *'in vivo' exposure* – that is actually exposing the patient to the stimulus that normally precipitates the compulsion, such as a dirty cloth in someone with compulsions relating to dirt and germs. There is less evidence that simply imagining the feared stimulus (*'imaginal exposure'*) rather than physically experiencing the feared stimulus is as effective
- it is more effective when the *therapist supervises* at least part of it rather than leaving it entirely to the patient to carry out (self-exposure)
- the patient must totally stop himself or herself from carrying out all aspects of the compulsion rather than allowing themselves to just reduce it. So-called *'total response prevention'* is required

- there is evidence that the *sessions need to be long enough* – probably longer than the characteristic hour-long sessions common in CBT (*see* Foa and Kozac, 1996).

Even after implementing the above conditions, there are problems with ERP. In particular, there are significant numbers of clients who refuse to undertake the exposure, in addition to significant rates of premature treatment termination (Stanley and Turner, 1995). Clark (2004) has suggested that this group who do not use ERP could benefit from *cognitive therapy* rather than more behavioural approaches. However, currently it is not proven that adding cognitive techniques generally improves the efficacy of ERP or that they are effective in clients who cannot use ERP (Clark, 2004; Heyman *et al*, 2006). There is evidence that CBT (including the cognitive elements) is effective for the treatment of *obsessive ruminations* without the overt compulsions (Freeston *et al*, 1997).

The review of the OCD outcome literature undertaken by NICE (2005a, see below) showed that the intensity of treatment (reflected in the number of hours of therapist input) predicted outcome. That is, patients who received more therapist input (over 10 hours) did better than those who received less input (fewer than 10 hours). There is also evidence that CBT delivered in a *group format* has equivalent outcomes for OCD compared to therapy delivered on an individual basis (McLean *et al*, 2001), and that these benefits are maintained at one-year follow-up (Braga *et al*, 2005). Recent evidence also points to equal effectiveness of CBT *delivered over the telephone* compared to face-to-face individual therapy (Lovell *et al*, 2006), although these results require replication.

NICE guidelines CG031: obsessive-compulsive disorder (NICE, 2005a)

These guidelines deal with both *OCD* and *body dysmorphic disorder* (BDD). They recommend differing treatments for mild, moderate and severe levels of functional impairment for adults with either disorder (they give separate recommendations for children, not covered by this book).

OCD in adults with mild functional impairment

The recommendation is to start with '*low-intensity psychological treatments*', particularly if the patient expresses a preference for such an approach. 'Low intensity' is defined as less than 10 hours' treatment per patient. It is important that a major component in each of these treatment modalities should be *exposure and response prevention* (ERP). Group therapy is defined as a low-intensity treatment. The three cited examples of low-intensity treatments are:

- individual CBT by telephone (C)
- structured self-help materials (C)
- group-delivered CBT (C).

When these prove inadequate or when the client cannot use them, then the recommended treatments are those cited under 'OCD in adults with moderate functional impairment' (C).

BDD in adults with mild functional impairment

'*Low-intensity*' psychological treatment is advocated (< 10 hours per patient) – this time individual or group-delivered CBT, which is tailored towards BDD and which again, includes ERP (B).

OCD in adults with moderate functional impairment

The psychological therapy recommended for this population is '*more intensive CBT*' (> 10 hours per patient that includes ERP), which should again incorporate ERP. The choice should be either this *or SSRI* medication, as the guidelines conclude that these treatments appear to be 'comparably efficacious' (B).

BDD in adults with moderate functional impairment

The guidelines again recommend the choice of *either* an *SSRI or* more *intensive CBT* (> 10 hours per patient that includes ERP), which addresses the key features of BDD (B).

OCD in adults with severe functional impairment

This time the recommendation is for *combined treatment* with more *intensive CBT and SSRI* medication (C).

BDD in adults with severe functional impairment

Again, the recommendation is *combined treatment* with more *intensive CBT* (> 10 hours per patient that includes ERP and which addresses the key features of BDD), *and SSRI* medication (C).

Further points

In addition to this staged approach to the treatment for adults with OCD/BDD the guidelines make the following general points:

- cognitive therapy in addition to ERP can be used to enhance the long-term reduction of symptoms (C)
- in some circumstances carers and family members can be used as co-therapists (B)
- CBT can be used where there are obsessive thoughts without overt compulsions (B)
- in some circumstances, such as when the client has severe functional impairment and is housebound, or when there is severe hoarding, then the client may need treatment at home (C). However, sometimes, for example when the hoarding prevents access, the treatment may need to be delivered by telephone (C)
- individual cognitive therapy should be considered when the client is unable or unwilling to use ERP (C)
- clients who request psychological therapies other than cognitive and behavioural approaches – such as psychoanalysis, hypnosis or couples therapy – should be told that there is *currently no convincing evidence* that they are effective treatments for OCD or BDD (C).

(Note also NICE 2006a – the Technology Appraisal 97: *Computerised Cognitive Behaviour Therapy for Depression and Anxiety*, which includes information about OCD and has been discussed earlier (p. 37)).

Post-traumatic stress disorder

Until relatively recently it was commonplace to offer single session 'debriefing' sessions immediately after and sometimes at the site of major disasters. This has changed after studies have generally shown this to be of no benefit or even detrimental (Sijbrandij *et al*, 2006). In contrast, there have been a significant number of trials that clearly show that *both CBT and EMDR (eye movement desensitisation and reprocessing) are efficacious treatments for post-traumatic stress disorder (PTSD)* (Foa *et al*, 2000; Bradley *et al*, 2005). These approaches have been shown to be 'highly effective'; in contrast, other approaches such as psychodynamic therapy and humanistic therapies have little evidence to support their worth in this disorder (Bradley *et al*, 2005). In a meta-analysis of 39 PTSD treatment studies, behaviour therapy, EMDR and antidepressant medication were found to be equally efficacious (van Etten and Taylor, 1998).

Generally the reviews show that exposing the patient to memories of what has happened is an essential part of treatment. That exposure can be to the literal place (in vivo exposure) or by remembering in detail what happened without actually being amongst literal reminders (imaginal exposure). More controversial points include:

- the extent to which adding *cognitive therapy elements* to the behavioural exposure adds significant benefit (Foa *et al*, 2003; Clark and Ehlers, 2004)
- whether all of the *elements of EMDR* are necessary. Specifically, whether the eye movement aspect of EMDR is necessary or whether the active part of EMDR is simply exposure to the memories (imaginal exposure) (Acierno *et al*, 1994)
- the *long-term efficacy* of psychological treatments for PTSD. It has not been clarified whether the lauded benefits of the CBT/EMDR approaches are maintained after a period of 12 months (Bradley *et al*, 2005)
- the role of EMDR and CBT in *childhood trauma*. Trauma sustained in childhood (particularly repeated trauma such as childhood abuse) can lead to different presentations compared with trauma that has only been experienced in adulthood. Those who have experienced childhood trauma are more likely to present with problems of impulse and emotional control, so that there is an overlap between conceptualising their problems as '*borderline personality disorder or traits*' and '*complex trauma*'. The potential benefit (and indeed risk) of using an exposure-based therapy in this group is controversial, and difficult questions remain in this frequently difficult-to-treat group (Bradley *et al*, 2005)
- the lack of *effectiveness* data. As already stated, the majority of research in psychological therapies is carried out in specialist centres not representative of the way treatment is delivered in routine settings (efficacy research). One of the minority of 'real-world' 'effectiveness' studies on PTSD observed the treatment of victims of the Omagh bomb in Northern Ireland (Gillespie *et al*, 2002).

NICE guidelines CG026: PTSD (NICE 2005b)

Initial response to trauma

- The NICE guidelines for PTSD clearly state that '*debriefing*', that is the provision of single-session interventions that focus on the recently experienced trauma, should *not* be routine practice (A).

- Rather, the guidelines suggest '*watchful waiting*' and the provision of a follow-up assessment after 1 month in those who present mild symptoms within 4 weeks of a trauma (C).

Trauma-focused psychological treatment

The treatment guidelines for PTSD provide differing advice depending on whether the disorder has been present for more than, or less than, three months' duration:
  In those who present within 3 months of the trauma the following apply:

1 *CBT (trauma–focused)* should be offered to those with PTSD within 3 months of the trauma (A), but within 1 month of the trauma if the PTSD symptoms are severe (B)
2 interventions that *do not focus on the trauma*, such as general relaxation techniques should not 'routinely' be provided (B)
3 the following are stipulated regarding the *form of the treatment* (grade B evidence):
  - it should last for 8–12 sessions (although fewer sessions may be needed if the patient is treated within the first month after the trauma)
  - longer sessions (e.g. 90 minutes) are usually needed if the trauma is the subject of the CBT session
  - the treatment needs to be provided on a regular (at least weekly) and continuous basis with the same therapist throughout treatment.

In those who present after 3 months, the treatment recommended differs in the following ways:

1 the recommended psychological therapy this time is *EMDR* as a potential alternative to *trauma-focused CBT* (A). The guidelines are clear that all PTSD patients should be offered one or the other, no matter how much time has elapsed since the trauma (B)
2 as for point 2 above (B), however this time the guidelines do say that if there has been no or only limited improvement with 'trauma-focused psychological therapy' then either *another form of trauma-focused psychological therapy* should be tried, or therapy should be augmented with *drug treatments* (C)
3 the same stipulated forms of therapy apply as described in point 3 above (B), but in addition the guidelines state that:
  - *12 sessions may not be enough* if one or more of the following apply (C) – when there has been not one but a number of traumatic events, when there has been a traumatic bereavement, when chronic disability has been a result of the trauma, where there are significant co-morbid disorders (such as depression or personality disorder), and when social problems are also present
  - sessions devoted to forming a *trusting relationship* and *emotional stabilisation* may need to occur before addressing the trauma *per se* in those patients who find disclosure of the trauma overwhelming (C).

Finally, the guidelines state that:

- there is *no convincing evidence* that other psychological therapies such as hypnotherapy or psychodynamic therapy have a 'clinically important effect' (GPP)

- when PTSD is co-morbid with *depression*, then generally the former should be treated first as the depression often improves when the PTSD gets better (C). However, the depression should be treated first when the psychological treatment of the PTSD would be seriously hindered by factors such as high suicide risk (C)
- when *drug or alcohol problems* might significantly interfere with treatment, then these need to be addressed first (C).

Schizophrenia and related psychoses

One of the drivers of research into psychological therapies for people with schizophrenia is the fact that so many continue to suffer from symptoms of psychosis (perhaps 40%) despite treatment with antipsychotics (Kane, 1996).

The finding that individuals with schizophrenia who reside in families with high 'expressed emotion' (EE) have higher rates of relapse than those in low-EE families (*see* Leff and Vaughn, 1985), has also spurred on research into family-based psychological treatments. These interventions vary in terms of the degree to which they merely educate the families (*psycho-education*), use *cognitive behavioural* approaches, and whether only one family is seen at a time or more than one (*multifamily group approach*) (Roth and Fonagy, 2005). The effects of these family interventions (at least in research centres) have been shown to be substantial. There are now meta-analyses that show reduced relapse rates that continue after the end of treatment (e.g. Pharoah *et al*, 2002), and reduced rates of readmission at two-years' follow-up (Pilling *et al*, 2002). One study carried out in the North West of England took a more formalised cognitive behavioural approach (Barrowclough *et al*, 1999). The relapse rates were about half in the CBT family intervention group relative to the 'standard care' group, although the overall admission rates of the two groups were not significantly different. It is important to note that the *delivery of services based on family-based psychological treatments* has not been as extensive as expected from the amount of supportive evidence. This may be because of the investment required to train people in the approaches and set up specialist services (Kuipers, 2000).

CBT delivered to patients on an individual basis has been investigated for community-representative samples of psychotic patients, for acute recent-onset psychosis, and for relapse prevention. More recently, studies have also begun to look at providing CBT interventions for people who are at very high risk of developing psychosis (Morrison *et al*, 2004). Although there is evidence that CBT can have significant benefits, once again *the evidence is not clear-cut*. A key issue is which outcome and which 'benefit' we deem important. Rector and Beck's (2001) meta-analysis of six studies investigating *CBT for delusions* found symptom benefits for CBT over and above less specific psychosocial interventions. Similarly, some individual studies have shown clear superiority of structured CBT-type approaches including in terms of re-admission rates (e.g. Bach and Hayes, 2002). However, other meta-analyses that have looked at relapse and re-admission rates have found that CBT does not reduce them relative to 'treatment as usual' (e.g. Pilling *et al*, 2002).

One well-known study into psychotic patients with a *mixed chronicity representative of CMHT caseloads* researched the effects of CBT delivered by community psychiatric nurses (CPNs) (Turkington *et al*, 2002). The effect of this additional treatment (over treatment as usual – TAU) was to reduce some symptoms such as depression, but the specific symptoms of schizophrenia were not significantly reduced. When the patients who had received CBT were followed up at one year, they had better insight into their condition, and had fewer negative symptoms and, importantly, had required significantly less time in hospital (Turkington *et al*, 2006). However, a major criticism of this study (and others in the field of psychosis) is that there was *no 'matching'* of the CBT and control patients in terms of the amount of face-to-face contact. It is therefore possible that the improvements were due to more personal care and contact rather than something specific about the delivered CBT *per se*.

Three trials for CBT for *acute-onset schizophrenia* have been by Drury *et al* (1996a, 1996b), Lewis *et al* (2002), and Startup and colleagues in North Wales (Startup *et al*, 2004, 2005). The first study showed very significant benefits from the CBT-based intervention compared to a control intervention. These included shorter hospital stays and faster recoveries from positive symptoms. However, the treatment given included individual, group and some family work. Roth and Fonagy (2005) point out that this means that the study does not prove effectiveness of individual CBT in that the family element may have been the 'active ingredient'. *Relapse rates were also no different* between the CBT and the control groups at 4-year follow-up (Drury *et al*, 2000). The study by Lewis and colleagues (2002) compared CBT, supportive counselling and treatment as usual. Their results showed no superiority of CBT compared to supportive counselling – only faster recovery in a subgroup suffering from auditory hallucinations at baseline. Eighteen months later, there was still no benefit from the CBT over counselling in terms of symptoms (although both groups did better than the controls). Results such as these have led some commentators to question whether the *specific intervention element of CBT* is necessary in the treatment of psychosis, or whether the more general human contact element is primarily active (Paley and Shapiro, 2002; Roth and Fonagy, 2005). Finally, the acute psychosis study by Startup and colleagues also showed superior improvement in symptoms with CBT. In this case the improvement was with hallucinations and delusions as well as negative symptoms and social functioning (Startup *et al*, 2004). However, two years later the CBT-treated patients were no better off in terms of positive symptoms compared to the TAU group (although they did have fewer negative symptoms and better social functioning) (Startup *et al*, 2005).

Other research has concentrated upon *relapse prevention* (e.g. Sensky *et al*, 2000; Gumley *et al*, 2003). Gumley and colleagues delivered variable doses of CBT dependent on the perceived risk of relapse. After one year, the CBT group had lower levels of symptoms but equivalent hospital admission rates to the TAU group.

Overall Roth and Fonagy (2005) conclude that *family interventions* do have an impact on rates of relapse. In comparison, *individually delivered CBT* in both the acutely ill (often first-onset) and the chronically ill generally appears to confer *benefits in terms of symptom relief* but not in terms of preventing episodes of relapse. Likewise, a Cochrane Collaboration meta-analysis concluded that CBT for schizophrenia may help symptoms over the medium term, but has not been shown to reduce relapse rates or re-admission compared to standard care (Jones *et al*, 2004). This remains a *controversial area*, with arguments passing backwards and forwards surrounding the adequacy of the evidence base, the applicability of the research to real-life services and whether CBT confers significant advantage over other intensive face-to-face professional contact (e.g Kingdon, 2006; McKenna, 2006). It is also an ethical argument in that some have argued that CBT can address issues such as *self-esteem, stigma, and attitude towards positive symptoms* – issues that are frequently neglected in routine care (Birchwood and Trower, 2006).

NICE guidelines CG001: schizophrenia (NICE, 2002)

The guidelines discuss the provision of psychological treatments for schizophrenia in two contexts – the early recovery time after the acute episode and later periods of illness where medication adherence and relapse prevention are themes.

Early post-acute period

A key theme here is the patient and family gaining a better understanding of the episode of illness that they have just experienced. The guidelines suggest the following:

- encouraging patients to write an account of their experiences of illness in their own clinical notes
- potentially using psychoanalytic and psychodynamic principles to help the health professionals understand their patients' experiences and relationships
- that *CBT is available* for patients with schizophrenia as a treatment option (A)
- the *provision of family interventions* for families who are in close contact with or who live with patients with schizophrenia (A)
- that supportive psychotherapy and counselling should not be routinely provided as 'discrete interventions' for people with schizophrenia when other psychological therapies have more evidence supporting their efficacy. Nevertheless, 'availability' and 'patient preference' are factors cited that might influence this (C).

Promoting recovery: relapse prevention and symptom reduction

The guidelines make the point that psychological therapies are now viewed as an essential treatment option that should be available to help the patient's (and the family's) recovery from schizophrenia, but that the *best evidence of efficacy is for CBT and family interventions*.

In terms of CBT the guidelines state:

- again, that CBT is a *treatment option that is made available* for people with schizophrenia (A)

but, in particular:

- CBT should be offered to those with persisting psychotic symptoms (A), and should be considered for those with poor treatment adherence (C) and to assist in the development of insight (B).

Longer treatments of CBT (more than 6 months and 10 planned session duration) are needed to change psychotic symptoms, shorter ones only really influencing depressive symptoms (A).

In terms of family interventions the guidelines recommend:

- providing family interventions for families who are in close contact with or who live with patients with schizophrenia (B)
- more specifically, CBT should be offered to families of schizophrenics who:
  - are considered at *risk of relapse* or who have *recently relapsed* (B)
  - have *persisting symptoms* (A).

Again, the guidelines recommend at least 6 months and 10 sessions of family intervention (A). They also recommend that, where practical, the patient should be present at the family sessions as this has been shown to improve outcome (A), while 'single family' rather than group 'multifamily' therapy may be preferred by patients and their families (B).

Eating disorders

The evidence base for the treatment of bulimia nervosa (BN; including CBT) is significantly better developed than the evidence base for the treatment of anorexia nervosa (*see* Palmer, 2004, 2006). There have been methodological problems in the research on anorexia. These have included the ethics of using a non-treatment control group in a potentially fatal disorder as well as the relatively high dropout rates from therapy. The latter reduces the power of studies to demonstrate a real difference between treatment options (Halmi *et al*, 2005). Yet, a few studies have shown benefit from *CBT in anorexia* (e.g. Pike *et al*, 2003), while other therapy models also have a limited evidence base supporting their use. For example, Dare *et al* (2001) found cognitive analytic therapy (CAT), focal psychodynamic therapy, and family therapy to be superior to 'standard care'. It is, however, unclear what the *active ingredients* are in psychotherapy for anorexia nervosa (AN). This has been recently illustrated by an RCT on 56 women comparing the structured approaches of CBT, IPT and non-specialised supportive psychotherapy (McIntosh *et al*, 2005). There was no apparent superiority of the CBT or IPT approaches over the supportive therapy; indeed, by some measures the non-specialised approach resulted in superior outcomes (the opposite of the researchers' initial hypotheses!). Yet, more studies have shown inconclusive results and even where there have been improvements, *relapse rates* at follow-up are high – up to 50% at one year (Pike, 1998). It is clear, therefore, that the current evidence base is not providing us with clear answers regarding the active ingredients in the psychological treatment of this difficult-to-treat disorder.

Meta-analyses show *large effect sizes for CBT in the treatment of bulimia nervosa* (BN; Thompson-Brenner *et al*, 2003). In common with AN though, many patients do not recover completely with therapy, and it has been noted that in the follow-up studies available, only 44% of clients meet the criteria for recovery at one year (Roth and Fonagy, 2005). An interesting pattern of outcomes has been observed with CBT, behaviour therapy (BT) and IPT in the treatment of BN (Fairburn *et al* 1991, 1995). In a group of 75 bulimics, those who received either BT or CBT initially did better than the IPT-treated patients. However, members of the BT group were more likely to both relapse and drop out of the trial, and the IPT group did better as the follow-up period progressed. Indeed, by 12 months the recovery rates for the IPT and CBT groups were not significantly different, while those of the BT group had fallen to less than half those of the IPT group. This pattern of improving IPT outcomes, referred to as an 'incubation' effect by Roth and Fonagy (2005), has since been replicated (Agras *et al*, 2000).

The *'stepped care'* models of treatment delivery for bulimia have also received limited evaluation. Treasure *et al* (1996) showed that bulimics who were offered a self-help manual as an initial step (only receiving subsequent one-to-one CBT if needed) had an equivalent outcome to those who automatically received one-to-one CBT. This is interesting, in that just less than one in three of the former group were so improved using the self-help that they did not need to have CBT with a therapist. It has been noted that self-help needs to be supported by some guidance from a worker to encourage compliance (Carter and Fairburn, 1998).

There is also limited evidence for the efficacy of *CBT in binge-eating disorder* (BED). Some researchers have again noted equivalent outcomes between IPT and CBT (Wilfley *et al*, 2002), and in common with bulimia, self-help can be effective when provided with some practitioner guidance (Carter and Fairburn, 1998).

NICE guidelines CG009: eating disorders (NICE, 2004c)

The NICE guidelines on eating disorders describe separately the treatment of AN, BN, and BED, but acknowledge that many patients have features of more than one of these and should be treated according to the disorder that their behaviour most closely resembles.

Anorexia nervosa

A common theme throughout the NICE guidelines for anorexia is the importance of *monitoring physical state including weight* alongside the psychological therapy. In response to the *poorer evidence base* for treatments in AN, NICE is less prescriptive about therapies to be used in anorexia compared to bulimia. It suggests that a number of psychological therapies can be considered, including CAT, CBT, IPT, focal psychodynamic therapy and family interventions that focus on eating disorders (C). The guidelines state that dietary counselling is inadequate as the only intervention for anorexia (C).

The guidelines recommend a number of *common elements* that should apply to all psychological treatments of anorexia nervosa:

- they should normally last for at least 6 months (C)
- the type of psychological therapy chosen should be influenced by the wishes of the patient and, where appropriate, the carer (C)
- there should be common therapy aims – to reduce risk, to encourage healthy eating and weight gain, to reduce other eating disorder symptoms and to assist with physical and psychological recovery (C)
- the professional needs to be competent and needs to be able to assess physical risk in therapy (C)
- if there is deterioration or no significant improvement during the time as an outpatient, then more intensive treatments (e.g. inpatient stay) need to be considered (C).

The guidelines provide recommendations about the psychological aspects of inpatient care for patients with anorexia:

- treatment should be structured, symptom focused and designed to achieve weight gain (C)
- there is a need to focus on wider psychosocial issues as well as eating behaviours and weight and shape, but there should be an expectation of weight gain (C)
- treatment should not comprise rigid behaviour-modification programmes (C)
- after weight restoration as an inpatient, outpatient follow-up should continue to focus not only on attitudes to weight, shape and eating behaviours, but also on *wider psychosocial issues*. There must continue to be regular *monitoring of psychological and physical risks* for at least *12 months post-discharge* (C).

Bulimia nervosa and binge-eating disorder

Key recommendations regarding the *treatment of bulimia* using psychological therapies are that:

- *CBT for bulimia (CBT-BN)* should be offered to adults with BN (16 to 20 sessions over 4–5 months are recommended) (A)
- if CBT is not successful or the patient doesn't want it, then the guidelines suggest *IPT* as an alternative (B), but state that patients need to be told that the evidence shows that IPT needs 8–12 months to achieve comparable results to those that CBT achieves in 4–5 months (B)
- a possible first step before one-to-one therapy is the use of *evidence-based self-help* (B), *supported* by a healthcare professional for improved outcome (B).

Finally, for BED, the guidelines are that:

- *CBT focused on BED (CBT-BED)* should be offered to adults (A). The duration of therapy and the required number of sessions are not specified
- *IPT and dialectical behaviour therapy* (DBT) may have a role with disorders that persist (B). However, all of the psychological treatments for BED have a *limited effect on body weight* (A), so that other treatments that specifically focus on *obesity* may also be required (C)
- the advice regarding *self-help* for BED (B), with *support* from a professional (B), is essentially the same as for bulimia.

Bipolar disorder

A key tenet of psychological treatments for bipolar disorder (BD) is that it is seen as an *adjunct rather than an alternative to medication* (Scott, 2001). The evidence base has developed greatly in the last five years, although there is still not the volume of research that there is for schizophrenia. The evidence base can also be somewhat confusing, in that there is a range of therapies all of which have similar aims of psychoeducation, stabilising mood through behaviour change and becoming aware of prodromes, and yet not all would class themselves as CBT. An example would be 'interpersonal and social rhythm therapy' (IPSRT) (Frank *et al*, 1999), which incorporates adapted IPT techniques. In one trial, IPSRT appeared to have a prophylactic effect, preventing new episodes in patients already diagnosed with bipolar I disorder (Frank *et al*, 2005). Similarly, family-based interventions have had some evaluation using similar treatment principles in addition to addressing high EE, as is the case in schizophrenia (e.g. Clarkin *et al*, 1990).

In terms of more formalised CBT for bipolar disorder, a number of RCTs have now shown a degree of superiority of CBT over standard care (e.g. Lam *et al*, 2003, 2005a; Scott *et al*, 2001, 2006a). Standard care referred to psychiatric follow-up in addition to medication such as mood stabilisers. Lam *et al* (2003) showed that patients prone to relapse who received CBT had 62 fewer days with bipolar episodes than the standard-care group over 12 months' follow-up. When the patients were followed up over 30 months after the end of therapy, they had 110 fewer days with bipolar episodes (Lam *et al*, 2005a). There was also a reduced rate of psychiatric inpatient admissions in the CBT group, who similarly adhered to their prescribed medication regime more than the control group. The benefits of the CBT continued for as long as two-and-a-half years post-treatment and were cost-effective (Lam *et al*, 2005b).

The findings of Lam and colleagues are somewhat at odds with a more recent significant multisite trial of 253 patients (Scott *et al*, 2006a). This used a very much more 'mixed' population of bipolar patients, including patients who were quite complex with co-existing substance misuse and more than one diagnosis. The results showed that CBT as an adjunct to medication and other treatments was only of significant benefit to those individuals who had had *12 or fewer episodes* of bipolar illness. These CBT recipients experienced fewer episodes of recurrence of illness over 18 months, compared to those who had not received CBT. The authors conclude that CBT should be predominantly used for those who are at an earlier stage of illness. They also acknowledge that their results were based on the delivery of 22 sessions of CBT, and that some more chronic and more complex patient presentations may benefit from more sessions of CBT (Scott *et al*, 2006b) – but this hypothesis has not been proven. CBT for bipolar disorder remains somewhat contentious and less researched than CBT for many other disorders.

NICE guidelines CG038: bipolar disorder (NICE, 2006b)

The guidelines come from a perspective that the treatment of bipolar disorder should be primarily medication based, but that psychological and psychosocial interventions also have a 'significant impact'. They describe a role for specific structured psychological interventions such as CBT. However, they also describe the important role of general advice in other settings such as promoting healthy lifestyles, regularity with routines, and sleep hygiene. This advice need not be given within a formal psychotherapy setting, although traditionally these have been elements of the CBT approach to bipolar disorder.

The guidelines recommend more formalised structured psychotherapy for bipolar disorder in the following circumstances (ratings for the strength of this supporting evidence were not available at the time of publication of this book):

- when there is an *incomplete response* to medication-based treatments for *acute depression*
- for *persistent depressive symptoms* – including for those who do not wish to take antidepressant medication

- in the *treatment of chronic and recurrent depressive symptoms* in combination with prophylactic medication (16–20 sessions)
- for people who are relatively stable but who may still have *mild/moderate affective symptoms* (16 sessions over 6–9 months) in addition to prophylactic medication. In terms of the specific areas covered by psychological therapies, the guidelines recommend the need to address the following:
  - medication concordance, psychoeducation and advice about daily routines and mood monitoring
  - detection of early-warning signs together with teaching strategies to prevent this progressing to 'full-blown' episodes
  - development of general strategies for coping
- in women who are *planning to become pregnant* who also become depressed after stopping prophylactic medication (CBT is specifically recommended)
- in *pregnant women* with mild depressive symptoms (the guidelines specifically recommend brief psychological interventions or self-help, including computerised CBT)
- in pregnant women with moderate-to-severe depressive symptoms. Here the guidelines specifically recommend CBT or combined medication with structured psychological intervention with severe depression.

The guidelines also state that there are roles for *befriending* and for *family interventions* that are outside the remit of this book.

Borderline personality disorder

The treatment of patients with borderline personality disorder (BPD) is complicated by:

- concerns over the validity of the diagnostic criteria
- *co-morbidity* with other mental health disorders. For example, over a period of one year more than half of a BPD patient population could also be diagnosed with GAD, and 40% had co-existing major depressive disorder (Swartz et al, 1990)
- complex *multifactorial aetiology* with clear links to complex childhood trauma
- *complex symptomalogy* including emotional dysregulation, psychotic symptoms and dissociative phenomena
- *high rates of morbidity and mortality.*

The most researched psychosocial interventions for patients with severe forms of this disorder are for *DBT* and *partial hospitalisation* (adapted from psychoanalytical psychotherapy; *see* Roth & Fonagy, 2005):

- *partial hospitalisation* has been shown to be effective in terms of reducing inpatient stays and suicide attempts. The improvements were maintained in many after 18 months and were cost-effective (Bateman and Fonagy, 1999, 2001, 2003). The effectiveness of intensive inpatient interventions has varied. One influential five-year study at the Cassel Hospital in London showed that patients with BPD did not benefit in this specialist unit any more than they did in standard psychiatric care (Rosser *et al*, 1987). A similar hospital in New York State appeared to show much better outcomes (Stone, 1993)

- *dialectical behaviour therapy* (DBT): Linehan initially evaluated this model for BPD and parasuicidal behaviour. A group who received DBT had a markedly reduced rate of hospital admission compared to a TAU group. The DBT patients were also less likely to engage in parasuicidal behaviour at six months' follow-up, although this advantage had disappeared by one-year follow-up after the treatment (Linehan *et al*, 1991, 1993). More recent work by Linehan has shown that one year of DBT input by 'experts' compared to equivalent hours of non-DBT input from other experts resulted in lower rates of parasuicidal behaviours in the DBT group. Indeed, the DBT group were half as likely to make suicide attempts and required fewer periods of hospitalisation. This indicates that there are specific elements of the DBT intervention that are beneficial in terms of reducing self-harming behaviours (Linehan *et al*, 2006). Nevertheless, the American Psychiatric Association (2001) points out that DBT is not proven with other aspects of BPD such as identity and interpersonal disturbances. There are now replications of Linehan's work, e.g. Verheul *et al* (2003)

- *schema-focused therapy* (SFT): the first schema-focused outcome study has recently completed in the Netherlands (Giesen-Bloo *et al*, 2006). At a number of sites, clients with BPD were randomised to either SFT or transference-focused therapy. SFT had superior outcomes in a number of variables, including anger reduction and emptiness, impulsivity and paranoid and dissociation scores. Both forms of therapy were provided weekly for three years. The researchers point out that DBT has not been shown to significantly influence these outcomes. They conclude, therefore, that DBT should be reserved for a subgroup of BPD clients with prominent parasuicidal behaviours (for which DBT does show efficacy)

- *more traditional CBT approach*: trials are beginning to emerge showing that the traditional CBT approach can improve outcomes for BPD. A well-known study is the *BOSCOT* trial based on 106 clients meeting a diagnosis for BPD (Davidson *et al*, 2006a, 2006b). The clients were randomised into a group who received CBT in addition to TAU, and another group who only received TAU. The trial was carried out in 'real clinic settings' rather than predominantly in a specialist academic environment. The CBT clients received an average of 16 sessions over a one-year period. This group had reduced rates of dysfunctional beliefs and reduced suicidal acts over the year of therapy and the subsequent year of follow-up. Although this is impressive, the CBT intervention did not bring about overall significant financial 'cost benefits' (Palmer *et al*, 2006).

MAIN POINTS

- CBT has a significant evidence base supporting its use in a range of mental disorders.
- NICE has published research-based clinical guidelines on the treatment of most mental disorders.
- Individual studies and meta-analyses support the use of CBT in depression.

- There is also increasing evidence supporting the use of computerised CBT programmes in depression.
- NICE guidelines support CBT as a treatment for depression, and as the psychological treatment of choice in moderate, severe, and treatment-resistant depression.
- Exposure-based behaviour therapy is efficacious for phobias, including agoraphobia and social phobia. There is also significant evidence supporting CBT for panic disorder.
- Antidepressant medication may assist CBT for panic, but benzodiazepines impair the outcome of exposure treatments in both panic disorders and phobias.
- There is less of an evidence base supporting the use of CBT for generalised anxiety disorder (GAD) – also just over 50% of treated clients show significant improvement (fewer than for other anxiety disorders).
- NICE guidelines recommend using CBT for panic disorder and GAD (including CBT-based self-help).
- Exposure and response prevention (ERP) is the CBT approach (and indeed the psychological approach) with the most evidence base for the treatment of OCD. There is also some evidence supporting the use of CBT delivered in groups to patients with OCD.
- Patients who have received CBT maintain more of the treatment gains than those who have received and then stopped clomipramine.
- CBT and eye movement desensitisation and reprocessing (EMDR) have been shown to be efficacious in the treatment of post-traumatic stress disorder (PTSD), and their adoption is recommended in the relevant NICE guidelines. 'Debriefing' is not recommended.
- Family approaches to the treatment of schizophrenia have an evidence base. These approaches often incorporate cognitive behavioural elements.
- There is evidence that one-to-one CBT for psychosis can significantly reduce symptoms.
- NICE guidelines on schizophrenia state that CBT should be available as a treatment option, and family interventions should be available to those in close contact with those suffering from schizophrenia.
- Both IPT and CBT have been shown to be effective for bulimia nervosa (BN). There is more of an evidence base supporting the use of all psychological therapies in BN than in anorexia nervosa (AN).
- NICE guidelines therefore state that IPT and CBT are the treatments of choice in BN, but are less prescriptive about the model to be adopted for AN.
- The evidence base for CBT in bipolar disorder is controversial, but currently shows that most patients can benefit – certainly those who have had fewer episodes of illness.
- CBT for borderline personality disorder is comparatively less researched. There is some evidence for a variety of psychological treatments including DBT, traditional CBT, schema-focused therapy and partial hospitalisation (based on psychoanalytic psychotherapy).

Further reading

- National Institute For Health and Clinical Excellence. nice.org.uk
- Roth A and Fonagy P (2005). *What works for Whom? A critical review of psychotherapy research* (2e). London: The Guilford Press.

Part 2

Doing it: the practice of cognitive behavioural therapy

Chapter 5

Taking a patient on for cognitive behavioural therapy

Chapter aims

- To consider the practical aspects of taking on a patient for CBT.
- To outline the cognitive behavioural assessment.
- To teach how to create a CBT formulation.
- To describe the basic structure of both a course of CBT and the individual sessions.

Can I start CBT with a patient?

You don't need to become an expert in CBT to help your patients using this approach.

Can you remember when you last tried to learn something new? It is probably worth *reflecting* on the process of what happened when you first started. The following questions can often help you (and your patients) to reflect:

- what went well?
- what didn't go so well?
- did you become good at it overnight?
- how did you improve?
- did you feel like giving up?
- who helped you succeed?

The answers to these questions will no doubt help you to consider whether some of your own anxious thoughts are appropriate or perhaps unhelpful. You will need to think about how much time you have to learn these skills so that your practice is safe and effective. You will need some specific targets to help you focus on what you will aim for and help you assess how you are doing. Traditionally we think of targets in three time scales:

- short term
- medium term
- long term.

Although there are no agreed definitions of these terms it is best to think of 'short term' as a few days, 'medium term' as a few weeks and 'longer term' as a few months or longer. What is important is that you have *clear goals* and devise a *structured plan* to attain them. All of us will have different agendas and circumstances. Some will want to become more involved with these CBT skills, others will want less. Some will want to tailor their skills to primary care, others to more specialised settings.

The point here is to think about your specific goals and be as effective as possible in achieving them.

Task 1: deciding upon your goal(s)

Spend 15 minutes thinking about your specific goals within the three time scales outlined above. Write them down.

You have just learnt your first CBT intervention: *goal setting*.

Task 2: can I achieve the goal(s) within the system in which I work?

Local systems in which we work will differ. When learning anything new we need to think about this system and how it could support our learning.

Spend 5 minutes thinking about the system where you work:

- who could supervise me?
- are any of my peers learning this new skill?
- what CBT resources are available to me?
- how much time will I have?
- when in my week can I do this? Maybe now isn't the best time
- how will I find a patient?
- what level of treatment will I use?
- how will I organise protected time?
- where will I see the patients?
- what will I learn from my sessions?
- will I audiotape or even videotape the sessions?
- how will I integrate my new skills into my subsequent clinical practice?

Task 3: problem solving – making a plan

Hopefully, after consideration you will have answers to the above questions. If not you might like to try to use a structured 'problem-solving' approach to do so.

Choose one of the above 'problems' or questions to be answered. We could for example try and work out who might supervise our practice. The problem could be defined as: 'I do not have anyone who could supervise me in CBT practice with patients'.

Once you are clear about the defined problem, six steps can be used to help you structure your response to it:

1 think up as many potential solutions as possible to overcome the problem

2   look at the advantages and disadvantages of each potential solution
3   choose one of the solutions
4   plan the steps needed to carry out that solution in as much detail as possible (include when and how you are going to do it)
5   carry out the plan
6   review the outcome.

Hopefully, this structure will assist you to develop and choose a specific plan to address the specific problem.

You have just learnt your second CBT intervention: *problem solving*.

If it helped you I wonder if it could help your patients?

I wonder if you could use any of these specific skills with a patient?

Things to know before your first case

Hopefully, you will now have specific goals and the beginnings of a plan for starting CBT in your work system. Before you send off your first appointment letter it is worth looking at an overview of a typical CBT treatment. We will describe the stages of therapy and related topics under the following headings:

- pre-assessment
- assessment
  - five-areas assessment
  - formulation
- structure of the therapy
- structure of the session
- supervision
- emotional aspects of ending

Pre-assessment

Finding the right first case is important

- What type of patient do you think would be suitable?
- How could you ensure you are referred one?

Designated CBT clinics are not that common, particularly in smaller centres. Therefore, patients are often seen by junior doctors for CBT within the setting of the CMHT or in outpatient clinics. In this environment it is likely that you will have to spend some time thinking carefully about which of the potential patients within the service might be suitable for CBT by a beginner. Advice from your supervisor is essential here. Your supervisor may be able to find you a case and will definitely be able to advise you about the suitability of one you may have in mind. Also it is important to request the mental health notes and to read them. Find out as much information as possible prior to sending out an appointment.

In order to decide who to choose, it would also be worth reading the paper 'Cognitive behaviour therapy for whom?' (Moorey, 1996, see Further reading, p. 86). In addition to the evidence base to support the use of CBT (or not support the use of CBT) for certain disorders, there are a number of other factors outlined by Moorey that influence outcome in CBT. These are as follows:

- *co-existing DSM-IV Axis I diagnoses*, such as depression in addition to OCD, may make treating either of the diagnoses using CBT more difficult or more time consuming
- *co-existing substance misuse*: as for the previous point, the treatment may become more complex and time consuming. In particular, benzodiazepine and alcohol misuse makes habituation less likely to happen with exposure for anxiety disorders. The substance misuse, therefore, usually has to be addressed first
- *co-existing DSM-IV Axis II diagnoses*: learning disability or personality disorder similarly can complicate therapy
- *the severity of the disorder*: generally more severe presentations are predictive of a poorer outcome, but not always
- *the chronicity of the disorder*: likewise, more chronic disorders usually have a poorer outcome
- *psychosocial factors such as ongoing severe stress or relationship problems*: if there are intractable background factors complicating the presentation, it stands to reason that the therapy is less likely to be effective
- *strong, fixed negative core beliefs (schemas) about themselves*: where this is the case, for example in patients with low self-esteem, the CBT may need to address the pre-existing belief system, in addition to treating the symptoms of the presenting problem
- *motivation for change*: some patients are more motivated than others to change their situation. A good example of this can be seen in patients with anorexia nervosa who may require significant time in therapy before feeling comfortable with trying out new eating behaviour patterns
- *ability to identify a clear goal for therapy*: better outcomes are generally achieved when patients are clear and specific about what they want to change. Aiming to reduce the frequency of a clearly defined behaviour is likely to be more achievable than a non-specific wish to just 'feel better'
- *ability to understand and work with the CBT model*: to some degree this relates to the general factor of *'psychological mindedness'*. This is the ability to stand back and reflect on your problems and think in a psychological way. Some patients, however, seem to specifically 'take to' the cognitive behavioural model, whereas others wish to explore underlying causes from their earlier lives. The latter may be better suited to a psychodynamic model of therapy
- *ability to complete homework tasks outside of the session*: this may relate to motivation. As the ability to generalise findings made in the session to life outside of the session is so crucial in CBT, the ability and willingness to complete homework tasks does predict how much benefit the patient is likely to get from the therapy.

The above pointers should be of assistance in choosing who is likely to benefit from CBT. It is particularly important for a trainee to select someone who is going to be relatively straightforward. As for *diagnostic problems* that are appropriate as an early case, it is the authors' opinion that a simple phobia or panic patient is perhaps most appropriate. Depression can be straightforward, although therapy for a case of severe depression should not be attempted. OCD and GAD can be difficult and probably should not be used as early training cases.

The initial appointment invitation letter

Patients are more likely to attend their appointment if you write an appropriate letter of invitation. The following are suggestions:

- personalise the letter by using their name: (Dear Mr/Miss/Mrs/Ms . . . surname)
- say *why* they are being contacted (*Dr X asked me to . . .*)
- outline *what* is being offered. For example say that it is an assessment appointment for cognitive behavioural psychotherapy
- outline any terms – such as the *meaning of CBT*. Many centres include written materials that describe in some detail what CBT is and how it works. It would be a good idea to *photocopy a short description of CBT* such as that outlined on the BABCP website (babcp.org.uk)
- further personalise the letter by commenting on the *general aims of therapy* in reference to their general clinical problem (*'can be helpful for problems of anxiety/depression/poor sleep'*)
- state how long the assessment appointment is likely to last for, who it will be with and the *purpose of the assessment itself* (i.e. assessment – *for us* to see if it may be helpful, *for them* to find out if treatment may benefit them)
- it is usually helpful to *attach directions* and perhaps a map and parking directions
- comment upon details for re-arranging the appointment if that is necessary, (*'if this is inconvenient please phone us at the above number and we will make all efforts to provide an alternative time for you'*)
- similarly, ask that they contact the department if they *decide not to attend* as someone else could use that appointment time
- it is encouraging to end with a statement such as: 'I look forward to meeting you', and then signing it personally.

Assessment and formulation

The purpose of the assessment interview(s) is to meet the patient in order to:

- let the patient tell their story
- allow the therapist to assess whether the patient is suitable for the treatment that *they are capable of offering*
- facilitate the patient's understanding of the treatment and therefore to . . .
- . . . facilitate the patient's ability to consent to that treatment.

This is going to involve:

- taking a *history* or *'screening interview'*
- completing a *mental state examination*
- making a *risk assessment*
- completing any *additional assessment tools* such as diagnostic inventories
- making a *diagnosis* (or diagnoses)
- constructing a *formulation*

- agreeing a *treatment plan* with the patient.

It is important to emphasise that your skills in taking a history, identifying risk and thinking laterally about other treatment approaches are as important as they are with all other patients. A common mistake is to concentrate heavily on the specific cognitive and behavioural model but to lose sight of the overall management of the patient. If, however, you wish to concentrate on the CBT, then it might not be unreasonable to ask someone else to see the patient separately for medication reviews. Some medically trained therapists do, nonetheless, manage to agenda this task into the CBT sessions. Although the subject of making a mental state examination and of making a risk assessment will not be addressed here, they should of course be an integral part of your ongoing contact with the patient, no matter what model of treatment is being used.

The cognitive behavioural screening interview

The term 'history' is less frequently used in CBT than in general psychiatry – the terms 'assessment' or 'screening interview' are more commonly used. However, the main function of information gathering in a structured way remains the same. The major cognitive behavioural elements of a cognitive behavioural history or screening are outlined in Box 5.1. It is important to integrate these questions into the history style that is already used by the clinician. For example, in the authors' opinion it is best for psychiatrists to add these themes to those of the standard psychiatric assessment (family history, personal history, psychiatric history, mental state examination, etc), rather than discounting this information that will help us in the overall management of the patient. It is also important to note that there will be *specific question areas that are particularly pertinent to different diagnoses*. So, for example, the issue of the 'body mass index' and influence of a distorted body image need to be addressed in patients with eating disorders. For this reason, each of the diagnostic areas addressed in Part 3 of this book has issues that need to be specifically addressed in assessment for CBT. *These questions should be asked in addition to rather than as an alternative to the question areas outlined in Box 5.1.*

Box 5.1 Question areas to be included in a cognitive behavioural history

(Note that questions specific to the diagnoses are outlined in Part 3 of this book)

1 What are the *presenting problems* (problem list)?
2 *Describe the problems in detail*: look for links and commonalities between the problems, e.g. their development over time, time of day, people who are present, where does it occur, how often, to what extent and for how long? This can be presented in the form of a *'behavioural analysis'* – i.e. *antecedents, behaviour* and *consequences*.
3 In anxiety disorders ask: *'What is the feared consequence?'* e.g. collapsing and having a heart attack in panic disorder.
4 Construct a *five-areas description* of the presenting problem(s) (see pp. 70–72) that connects them, noting patterns of:
   - altered thinking (NB cognitive distortions)

   – altered behaviours
   – altered physical symptoms
   – altered mood/ emotions.
5 Describe how each of the areas of the five-areas model influence each other during a discrete period of time (*modulating factors*): e.g. the influence of being tired on patterns of thinking.
6 Would the features in the five-areas model have been worse if some factors had not been present (*protective factors*): e.g. a supportive partner?
7 How have the five areas continued over time, i.e. what is keeping the problem going (*maintaining factors*)? NB look out for *avoidance and safety behaviours.*
8 Previous *attempts to treat* the problem: these may be professional, e.g. previous therapy, or non-professional, e.g. illicit drug use. *What effect* did these treatments have?
9 What have been the *effects of the problem(s)*: e.g. loss of job?
10 What is the *patient's understanding* of the problem(s) and the treatment that they hope/expect will alleviate it (them)?
11 What is the *patient's capacity* to use CBT (socialise to model)?

As in the usual psychiatric history the cognitive behavioural screening assessment begins with an enquiry into the patient's current problem(s). Some clinicians work together with the patient to construct a *problem list* (Persons, 1989). This list can then be looked at to see if the discrete problems are actually linked, thus displaying an underlying problem that in itself needs to be addressed. For example, a problem with a partner, friend and debt may point to a problem with assertiveness that can be addressed as an issue in its own right.

The problems need to be *described in detail* – what, when, how, who, etc. This description will help to point to common causes.

Then the major problem or problems can be split up into associated moods, behaviours, thoughts, and physical symptoms. This helps us to construct a *five-areas assessment* (Williams, 2001) of the problem. While doing this it is useful to note characteristic unhelpful thinking styles (cognitive distortions). The five-areas assessment is the first step towards constructing a five-areas formulation as described later in this chapter.

The next step towards this formulation is to assess how all of the areas within the five-areas model *influence each other* during important periods. For example, during a panic attack, how does the situation that the patient is in influence their thoughts? In turn how do these influence the physical symptoms, and how are these interpreted to influence their behaviour and so on. These influences over a discrete period are known as modulating factors. For example, being in a city centre may '*modulate*' the likelihood of thoughts that others are looking at you in a disapproving way, or tiredness may modulate whether cognitions with a cata-strophic content are experienced or not. Over the longer term, some factors have an influence not just on the degree to which a problem is manifest at a given time but also on whether the problem continues over the longer term. These factors are known as '*maintenance factors*'. In the CBT model we are particularly interested in *safety behaviours* and patterns of *avoidance* that can serve to maintain the underlying problem.

It is important not to simply look at the pathology, at what is wrong, but to also look at what is right. This is hugely important, but often does not come naturally to doctors who are used to concentrating on pathology and diagnoses. Some patients cope well in certain key ways. Others have protective relationships or other situations such as a fulfilling job that protect them. These can be amplified in treatment to assist better management of the problem(s). So we need to assess positive coping strategies and *protective factors* fully.

We need to know how the patient has tried to treat the problem in the past (professionally or otherwise), and the effect of these attempts. We need to know how they view their problem – what name they give it and how they believe it should be treated. This will give us clues as to the appropriateness of CBT and the patient's ability or capacity to use the treatment model. The aforementioned factors that are known to influence outcome in CBT (Moorey, 1996) will influence this decision.

Another way in which we can assess the ability to use the model is to '*socialise the patient to the model*'. This simply refers to the task of presenting the CBT model to the patient (general model or the specific model for the disorder), and allowing the patient to incorporate the specifics of their situation into this model. If the patient is able to understand and relate to the model, then they are obviously more likely to be able to work with it in subsequent treatment sessions. Where they are not able to see the relevance but prefer to understand the issues along more pharmacological lines, then we may decide not to embark on formal CBT but to prescribe instead. Alternatively, of course, we may decide to do both.

Self-report and interview questionnaires

Rating scales are used extensively in CBT. This is particularly the case in the assessment process where questionnaires such as the Beck Depression Inventory (version II) (BDI-II) (Beck *et al*, 1996) and the Beck Anxiety Inventory (BAI) (Beck *et al*, 1988) are used by a large proportion of CBT therapists. These questionnaires are completed by the patient and are thus known as self-report measures. Rating scales are available for almost all problem areas, and are increasingly used in all clinical work, not just CBT. It is outside the remit of this book to describe the array of questionnaires now available. Some rating scales have a predominant CBT focus by asking questions mainly about cognitions and behaviours (e.g. Hopelessness Scale, Beck *et al*, 1974). Others such as the Clinical Outcomes in Routine Evaluation rating scale (CORE) (*see* Barkham *et al*, 1998) and the Health of the Nation Outcome Scale (HoNOS) (*see* Wing *et al*, 1998) are used throughout British mental health services and not predominantly within CBT settings. Currently there is debate about which of these measures most accurately capture the most relevant outcomes in mental health (e.g. Leach *et al*, 2005). The main reasons why rating scales are so often used in CBT include the following:

- they allow the therapist to compare the status of the patient pre-treatment and post-treatment to assess the effectiveness of the intervention for that particular patient

- by compiling the pre–post questionnaire data for each of the patients we can deduce an estimation of effectiveness of the department as a whole. These data can then be compared with compiled effectiveness data from other treatment centres. This process is called *'benchmarking'*. Its aim is to compare treatment methods, and to subsequently adopt methods that appear to be particularly effective in some centres, in order that treatments can be improved
- they are used in *research* including in RCTs to compare the efficacy/effectiveness of different interventions
- they help the *initial clinical assessment*, by indicating the severity of the different problem areas and the related functional impairment. However, self-report measures should not be considered equal to a full face-to-face clinical assessment with mental state examination
- sometimes rating scales are completed at a number of *points throughout therapy*, to assess the effectiveness of discrete interventions within therapy
- occasionally, the rating scale is completed because the *topic area is specialised* and it would not routinely be assessed in an interview. This may be the case for the Dysfunctional Attitude Scale (DAS) (Weissman and Beck, 1978). This questionnaire allows the client to indicate how they would respond to varying life scenarios.

As can be seen, the procedure of assessment for CBT is made up of a lot more than choosing an ICD-10 (International Classification of Disease) or DSM-IV (*Diagnostic and Statistical Manual of Mental Disorders*) diagnosis. Although it is essential to make a diagnosis, doing so is not going to individualise a *treatment plan*. Only by constructing a formulation will we be able to devise a treatment plan to direct the way forward through therapy.

Writing a CBT formulation

A cognitive behavioural formulation is an individual explanation of the patient's difficulties, using a CBT theoretical model. This will inform treatment. Chapter 3 of this book outlines how a formulation is usually constructed in general psychiatry and how the emphasis changes between theoretical models. In common with all aspects of CBT, there is agreement that the process of arriving at a cognitive behavioural formulation is not done by the therapist or the patient alone but in *collaboration*. It is openly discussed and is an active piece of joint working, which will change as more information becomes available. This may be the case at any point throughout treatment.

When starting out in this approach it is best to keep it simple. The skills involved in producing a cognitive behavioural formulation are a lifelong learning exercise. It is best remembered that *the formulation is a way to describe and simplify a very complex system, and its purpose is to inform decisions on how to proceed*. It ties theory to treatment for the individual patient. It does not need to include all the relevant information – only that which directly helps with this general purpose.

When forming an initial clinical impression of a patient, it may be useful to start by constructing a general psychiatric formulation – thinking in terms of three types of causal factors: 'predisposing', 'precipitating' and 'maintaining' (sometimes the word 'perpetuating' is used to make three 'P's!). This is described in Chapter 3. The example used was Edward, a 21 year old with symptoms of psychosis. Later in this chapter we use another example – Sadie, a 52-year-old woman who has been referred for CBT for moderate depression.

Although the *general psychiatric formulation* (the *three 'P's formulation*) is useful, it does not really look at the relationship between thoughts, feelings and behaviours. A more helpful assessment model would also concentrate on these aspects of the human condition (certainly for any CBT work). A reasonable initial step towards constructing a detailed cognitive behavioural formulation is to create what is known as a *five-areas formulation* (Williams, 2001). This formulation is easily worked out collaboratively with the patient. It can serve to describe the relationships between the patient's thinking, physical symptoms, moods/emotions, and behaviours. In addition it can also be used to describe or *'socialise' the cognitive behavioural model* to the patient.

Constructing a five-areas formulation (Williams, 2001)

A five-areas formulation is founded on a relatively simple assessment based mainly on the patient's situation and functioning *'in the here and now'* (rather than a detailed exploration of past events). It aims to divide up the problems that the patient presents with into 'areas' of 'altered thinking', 'altered emotional feelings and moods', 'altered behaviours', 'altered physical feelings', and finally 'life, situation, relationship, or practical problems'. The model itself is shown in Figure 5.1, whilst an example of a five-areas formulation is shown in Figure 5.2 for 'Sadie' – whose history is outlined later in this chapter. The process of dividing up the presenting features into these separate areas helps the patient to break down their problems and to begin to see the relationships between them. For example, they may begin to see that a negative thought has an effect on their mood, or on their behaviours. It will also enable treatment to be directed to specific issues. As *each area relates to all the others*, change in one will influence the others (the reason why there are two-headed arrows!). Therefore, in many ways it does not matter where on the diagram we start to describe the current situation to the patient – it does not have to be at the top! For example, if we were to prescribe an SSRI antidepressant medication it is likely to have an effect on all of the areas. This physical treatment would alter the brain's neurochemistry, which might alter the biological symptoms of depression described under 'altered physical feelings' (e.g. by improving impaired sleep or appetite). We may therefore start in this 'physical feeling' area and look at the resulting effects in the other areas. For example, it may allow the patient to engage again in more pleasurable activities, with a resulting benefit in the way they think about themselves and an improving mood state. It helps if the initial assessment asks for the features in the five areas separately, in order to complete a five-areas assessment. This can be refined later with an exploration of how the five areas influence each other. This then forms a five-areas formulation.

Alternatively, we could present the same information in the form of a *'behavioural analysis'* where there is identifiable problem behaviour. This sets out the most important factors over time in the form of *'ABC'*, that is the *'antecedents'* that predict the unhelpful behaviour, the *'behaviour'* itself, and then the *'consequences'* of that unhelpful behaviour. For example, a patient referred with aggression on a hospital ward may exhibit a 'problem behaviour' in the evening after dinner when the ward is quiet and the patients are resting. The consequences of the behaviour might be

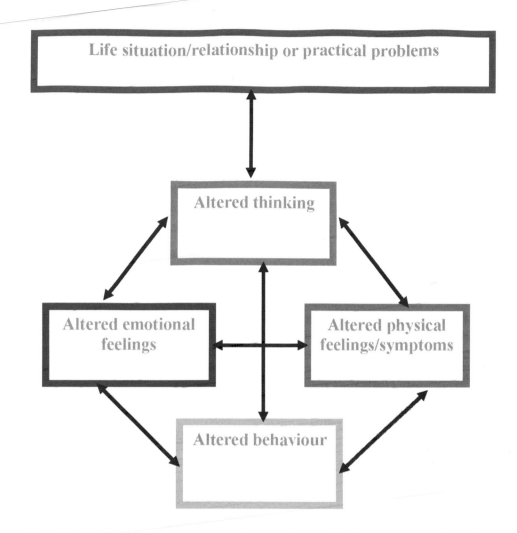

Figure 5.1 The five-areas assessment and formulation model (from *Overcoming Depression: a five areas approach* © Dr CJ Williams (2001) Reproduced with permission of Edward Arnold (Publishers) Ltd.)

that the ward staff go over to the patient and give lots of attention. This behavioural analysis may point to changes in the behaviour of the ward staff required to 'extinguish' the unhelpful behaviour of the patient. This could also be presented as a type of formulation – particularly if there is an attempt to explain the connections between A, B, and C using cognitive behavioural principles. This book, however, concentrates on the five-areas approach as the major basic way of formulating a case.

It is the ability to produce a formulation that enables problems to be specifically targeted and treated. This simple cognitive behavioural therapy formulation will start the patient thinking about unhelpful thoughts and behaviours. However, to understand more we have to add more complexity.

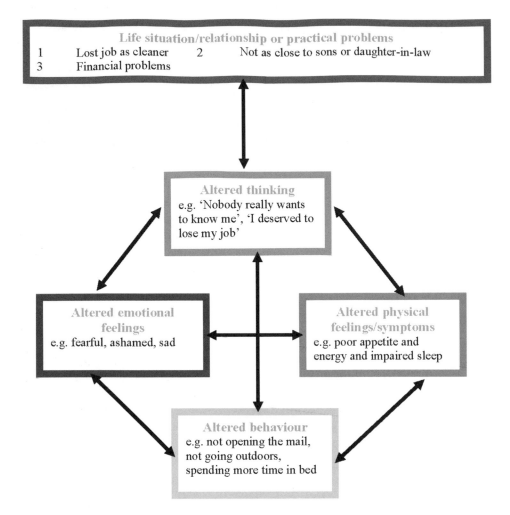

Figure 5.2 Example of a five-areas formulation for Sadie – a 52 year old woman with depression (from *Overcoming Depression: a five areas approach* © Dr CJ Williams (2001) Reproduced with permission of Edward Arnold (Publishers) Ltd.)

Constructing a 'linear' CBT formulation

The formulation should help us answer the following questions:

- why has the patient developed these symptoms now?
- what keeps them going?
- how do you understand or make sense of it?
- what do you think is going on?
- how does this all fit together?
- what might be the missing links?
- is there a pattern here?
- what is going well?
- what is not going well?

Box 5.2   Some definitions

Assumption
This is the act of taking something for granted, or supposing something without proof or based on incomplete evidence.

Cognition
The psychological result of perception, learning and reasoning. The most common forms of cognition are thoughts, other forms are images and belief structures.

In CBT theory, early experiences shape our *beliefs* and *assumptions*. We all have many underlying assumptions. These can develop in helpful ways and provide meaning and understanding, which can be used to assess the present and to prejudge the future. We have assumptions about behaviour, thoughts, emotional experiences, and relationships. At times these core beliefs and assumptions are unhelpful, leading to more unhelpful thoughts that produce unhelpful behaviours and feelings. These can produce *vicious circles* of thoughts, behaviours and feelings, which become the symptoms of mental illness. In treatment, we are most interested in identifying the underlying assumptions that maintain problems and helping our patients understand the implications of holding on to these.

A linear CBT model would include *Beck's model of depression* (Beck *et al*, 1979). Beck stated that early experiences such as neglect, as well as biological factors such as a genetic predisposition to depression, form a vulnerability to becoming depressed in later life. These early life experiences also result in the development of related *core beliefs* (sometimes called *schemas*) and *basic assumptions* – described in Chapter 7. These are basic beliefs and rules through which we see the world and interpret events. We all hold them – they are necessary to structure perception; however, if our early experiences are particularly challenging, then our core beliefs and assumptions can become negatively influenced by these experiences. For example, a neglectful or emotionally abusive childhood can cause the affected person to form a core belief about themselves as 'worthless' or 'stupid'. They may believe a rule or basic assumption that: 'if I give too much information about myself to others then they'll reject me'. Beck said that although these beliefs and assumptions are generally formed early in life, they might not be that influential until a key life event in later life *activates* them. For example, someone with a core belief that: 'I am worthless' and a basic assumption that: 'if I give too much information about myself to others then they'll reject me' may be hugely affected by a relationship breakdown. The result in this case might be that the person starts to blame themselves for the relationship breakdown – 'who would want to go out with me anyway?', 'I suppose it was going to happen sooner or later', 'I'll always be on my own – what's the point in trying to meet anyone else?' These last statements (reflecting thoughts) pop into the person's head readily, but their content can be understood in the context of the activated core beliefs and the assumptions. Because of the way they pop into our consciousness and their negative content they are called *'negative automatic thoughts'* (NATs). Beck said that it is this tirade of negative automatic thoughts that can be seen in sufferers with depression and which act as a maintaining factor for the depression itself. Note that NATs are usually written down in speech marks as if the person had just said the thought – rather than the therapist's description about the rough content of the thinking. Likewise core beliefs are written down as: 'I am . . .' statements or sometimes as 'others are . . .' statements. Basic assumptions or rules are usually written down as the exact rule – normally: 'If . . . then . . .' statements or sometimes as: 'I must . . .' or 'I should . . .' statements.

The effect of these NATs is frequently to cause the person's mood to drop (altered emotional feeling) or for their behaviours to change (altered behaviour), and sometimes they influence physical symptoms such as tiredness. Therefore, we can

Early experiences and biological factors
(predisposing factors forming psychological vulnerability)

↓

Development of basic assumptions and core beliefs
'I am . . .'
'They are . . .'
'The world is . . .'
'If . . ., then . . .'
'If I don't . . . then . . .'
'I should . . .'

↓

Critical incident or situation
(precipitating factors to the problem)

↓

Basic assumptions and core belief activated

↓

Negative automatic thoughts (NATs)
(maintaining factors to the problem)
(this can be used as 'altered thinking' area in five-areas formulation)

↓

Other areas of the five areas formulation
(altered emotional feelings, altered behaviour, altered physical feelings/symptoms)

Figure 5.3 The 'linear' CBT formulation (based on Beck *et al*, 1979).

add the five-areas formulation to the end of the linear description of the formation of the underlying core beliefs and assumptions. This 'linear'-type formulation can form the basis of a formulation to guide treatment when you see someone for depression; however, it can also be useful in understanding other conditions. For example, a social phobic patient may have been bullied in childhood, resulting in the development of core beliefs that: 'I am stupid' and 'I am defective'. The resulting assumption may be: 'if I show my real self in front of people they will humiliate me'. A critical incident may be a relationship breakdown or a perceived humiliation event in front of a group of people. This activates the assumptions and core beliefs resulting in NATs about how 'others must be laughing at me', how 'nobody will want to see me this Christmas', and many more similar NATs with the same theme. We can then map the remaining three areas of a five-areas formulation at the end of the linear formulation with the NATs forming the 'altered thinking' area (*see* Figure 5.3). Predictably, the altered behaviour includes avoidance of contact with others and the altered physical symptoms include increased agitation and poor sleep. The patient's predominant altered emotional feeling may be of shame. You can see, therefore, how this linear formulation can be useful for understanding the presentation of many patients, particularly when you include a five-areas understanding of their current functioning. Within exam situations (e.g. part II membership exams) it may be best to stick to this linear formulation or a basic five-areas formulation rather than attempting a formulation based upon the specific CBT model for that specific disorder.

Example of the assessment and formulation process

Box 5.3   Summary of screening interview, mental state assessment, risk assessment and rating scales

A 52-year-old woman called Sadie was referred by her GP for CBT for moderate depression. She had most symptoms of a depressive episode including poor concentration, poor motivation, low energy levels and tearfulness (*presenting problems*). Sadie had always been anxious and had always worried about how she looked to others. Although she believed that she had been low in mood for 2–3 years, her situation had deteriorated after she was made redundant from her job as a hospital cleaner seven months previously. At the time that she lost her job she felt very ashamed and to some extent blamed herself. She said that 'deep down' she always viewed herself as 'useless' – a view that was reinforced by her mother who used that term throughout Sadie's childhood. Sadie's mother had also suffered with 'nerves' but has never been depressed. Sadie has two sons, a daughter-in-law with whom she has traditionally been quite close and a small number of good friends and neighbours who have always meant a lot to Sadie. She believes that they don't really want to know her now, and that when they try and contact her that they are 'only doing their duty'. When she sits she thinks over and over about this and she becomes tearful and lower in her mood (ruminating as a *moderating factor*). In the last 6 weeks she has stopped answering telephone calls and no longer opens her mail. This has led to a worsening situation with Sadie's finances – as she is not responding to her creditors. This in turn appears to have led to a general deterioration in Sadie's mood and physical symptoms of depression (*maintaining factors*). When her daughter-in-law has tried to sort this out Sadie has been reluctant to admit that there is a problem. Sadie has stopped going outdoors for two months and spends her time sitting watching TV (*maintaining factor?*). She cannot say, however, what she has watched. She does believe herself to be ill, but does not believe that she can help herself as she had tried St John's wort, which did not help. She wanted to try CBT after having read an article in a newspaper supplement. She grasped the main concepts involved in the CBT model of depression after she was *socialised to the model* and was very *motivated* to try things out at home. She appeared to have the *capacity* to use the model and was judged to be suitable for CBT treatment. This decision was also based on the *risk assessment* and *mental state examination* that indicated that it was safe to offer CBT treatment as an outpatient. Just prior to the assessment interview Sadie completed the *Beck Depression Inventory – version II (BDI-II)* (Beck *et al*, 1996) which gave a score of 26. This indicated 'moderate depression'. Importantly on the item in the BDI-II that assesses suicidal ideation she had responded that she was not having thoughts of wanting to 'kill herself'. The *Beck Anxiety Scale* (BAI) (Beck *et al*, 1988) gave a score of 17, indicating 'moderate anxiety'.

Diagnoses
- Recurrent depressive illness, current episode moderate
- Some symptoms of agoraphobia
- (In addition Sadie probably had low self-esteem that pre-dated the depressive episode).

Three 'P's formulation
- Predisposing factors:
  - biological predisposition to anxiety?
  - tendency in the past to use avoidance as predominant coping strategy
  - viewed self from early age as 'useless' – note relationship with mother
  - shy and introverted
- Precipitating factors:
  - loss of her job
- Maintaining factors:
  - avoiding going out
  - avoiding opening mail with resulting practical problems – especially the debt
  - worrying about how she is thought of by others
  - social isolation
  - financial threat.

'Five-areas' assessment (see Figure 5.2)
- Life situation/relationship or practical problems:
  - poor relationship with mother

- lost job as cleaner
- not as close to sons or daughter-in-law
- little contact with others
- Altered thinking:
  - 'nobody really wants to know me'
  - 'if I went out people would think I looked odd'
  - 'I deserved to lose my job'
  - 'I'm worthless'
  - 'why do I bother?'
  - 'if I try and call up my old friends they won't want to know'
  - 'I'm safe now only if I stay indoors'
  - 'the future holds no joy for me'
  - 'the mail is going to tell me something that I just can't cope with hearing'
  - 'I must be an embarrassment to my sons'
- Altered feelings:
  - anxious
  - sad
  - fearful
  - ashamed
- Altered physical symptoms:
  - poor concentration
  - poor appetite
  - little energy
  - no motivation
- Altered behaviours:
  - not answering phone
  - not opening the mail
  - not going outdoors
  - spending more time in bed
  - not cooking or cleaning.

Extended 'linear' CBT formulation

- Early experiences and biological factors:
  - attacked by mother verbally on regular basis as a child
  - anxious mother
  - shy
- Development of core beliefs:
  - 'I'm useless'
  - 'I'm vulnerable'
  - 'the world is dangerous'
- Development of basic assumptions:
  - 'if you appear vulnerable then others will attack you'
  - 'if people see how useless I am then they'll reject me'
  - 'if people knew the "real me" they would be ashamed of me'
  - 'my worth is dependent on what I can do for others'
- Critical incident or situation:
  - made redundant from her job as a cleaner

- Unhelpful thoughts:
  - 'I'm ashamed to go out'
  - 'I will be polite to my friends but not bother them with my problems'
  - 'I don't want to "put on" my friends or they will drift away from me'
  - 'I need to keep my problems from my sons – they have enough to deal with'
  - 'if my sons knew what I was going through then they'd be angry with me'
- Impact of unhelpful thoughts:
- **Positive impact**
  - nil – her family and friends worry *more* not less when Sadie hides away and refuses to talk
- **Negative impact**
  - no contact with friends who were an important part of Sadie's life and who used to give her pleasure when she met them
  - anxious when thinking about going out, so she stays indoors
  - not able to talk with family (or friends) about how she feels
  - friends and family feel guilty that they have 'wronged' Sadie in some way and at times have started to avoid her
  - Sadie is unable to test whether her unhelpful thoughts are valid.

Example of a 'vicious circle' maintaining Sadie's problems (this could be used to 'socialise' Sadie to the CBT model')

Situation

10:30 am Sadie's neighbour calls to ask if she would like to attend church that evening.

Thoughts

- 'She thinks I'm a "basket-case" – she's just being polite.'
- 'She really wants me to say no – she can't really want me to go with her.'
- 'If Josephine knew what I was like really, then she'd be appalled and not want to know me any more.'
- 'I need to hide what is happening from Josephine.'

Feelings

- Ashamed
- Low

Behaviours

Sadie says she no longer enjoys church. She has little eye contact with Josephine when she talks with her.

Outcome

Sadie's neighbour believes her story and thinks that she is 'intruding on Sadie'. She decides to leave it to Sadie to contact her next, so does not visit the following week.

Thoughts

Sadie interprets the lack of a visit the following week as evidence that Josephine does not think that Sadie is 'worth bothering with'. This reinforces her belief that she is useless and she is even less likely to contact others therefore completing the vicious circle.

Key points

The core belief: 'I'm useless'

Sadie has held this belief to some degree since childhood – it is understandable that she holds the belief because her mother repeated it to Sadie as a child. What is important here is that the *critical incident* of the redundancy *reactivated* this core belief. New events would therefore now be more likely to be interpreted in the context of holding this belief about herself.

The assumption: 'if people really knew me then they would reject me'

It can be seen how this assumption is understandable in the context of Sadie's childhood, and core belief of: 'I'm useless'. However, it is also an assumption that could be tested in some way – perhaps it is only partially true or not true at all. We have to ask what impact holding this assumption is having on Josephine's life.

The unhelpful thought: 'I need to hide what is happening to me from Josephine'

The assumption: *'if people really knew me then they would reject me'* is implicated in the production of this unhelpful thought. What does Sadie really believe Josephine is going to think and do in response to her admitting that she is struggling with depression? Perhaps this could be tested? There are probably advantages and disadvantages to the resulting behaviour of hiding information from Josephine. Sadie hasn't had to explain what is going on, which might prove difficult, but she has also been left without support and without support to help her to church – a Sunday evening activity that Sadie previously enjoyed and valued very much.

The impact of these unhelpful thoughts, assumptions and beliefs

What is the price of these thoughts for Sadie? One is the reinforcement of her own belief that she is useless. The misinterpretation of the behaviours and words of others 'prove' this for Sadie. There will be further deterioration in her mood, and other unpleasant feelings. Sadie may engage in further unhelpful behaviours and may lose friendships, all leading to a deterioration of her symptoms of depression (including the biological ones). It is the assumptions and unhelpful thoughts and behaviours that are causing the difficulties and probably maintaining the depression.

Over the course of treatment, more information may become available and the above formulation may change. The last remaining step for Sadie once she has entered therapy, been assessed and a formulation created, is to decide upon the goals for treatment and finally to agree upon a general treatment plan.

When Sadie did agree to come for CBT she agreed the following *goals* with the therapist:

- to be able to 'understand' what was happening to her
- to start to attend church again
- to sleep more than her current 4 hours per night
- to feel better in her mood.

These goals may appear achievable but Sadie and her therapist need to make changes to allow them to happen. Our *formulation* will help point us to the changes that need to be made and the *CBT techniques* outlined in the next chapter will help to put those changes into practice.

The structure of the therapy

So you have now developed an initial formulation with the patient. A decision has to be made about whether the patient will benefit from treatment. Not everyone is suitable for CBT, or indeed would choose to receive this model of therapy. So, as with any treatment, the patient has to give informed consent. He or she needs to hear about the structure and time course of the treatment, its benefits and side-effects and the likely effect of not having CBT.

DSM-IV (American Psychiatric Association, 1994) separates mental disorders into Axis I and Axis II disorders. Axis I refers to mental illness and Axis II refers to learning difficulties and personality disorders. For most DSM-IV Axis I disorders (such as depression, GAD or OCD) with moderate complexity, a treatment course of *between 10 and 20 hourly sessions over 6 months* would be about right. Seeing the patient weekly at the beginning and then spacing out towards the end with a review session one month after completing treatment is common practice. Being *explicit about the likely time course* is also good clinical practice. At the beginning of treatment the patient and therapist usually agree upon the number of sessions that will be provided. This is sometimes referred to as '*setting a contract*'. Initially contracting for four or six sessions and then reviewing progress at that point is another frequent model of contracting. This sets the tone for the expectation of progress and commitment to change. It is the therapist's responsibility to set *agreed boundaries* for the treatment. These vary to some degree but will normally include an expectation that both the therapist and patient turn up for appointments on time and will contact each other if either is not able to attend. There will often be clear agreed boundaries on contact between the patient and the therapist outside of the sessions, for example in *periods of crisis*. If the therapist is not to provide crisis interventions then it may be necessary to consider which organisation will do so if there are issues of risk. A particularly important issue is the consideration of who takes ultimate clinical responsibility for the patient. The *CBT supervisor* may take responsibility for the CBT supervision but the medical responsibility (sometimes referred to as '*RMO responsibility*') may need to continue to lie with the CMHT psychiatrist – consider risk and who will assess and provide inpatient facilities if there is a problem. Simply being a psychiatric trainee also infers a need for a senior psychiatrist to take clinical responsibility for the patient's overall care. All of these boundaries will need to be considered and explicitly agreed upon before treatment can proceed. Some centres write out a *written contract* and ask the patient and therapist to sign it. In some ways these issues are particularly important to consider for the junior psychiatrist, as the frequency of contact and the personal nature of some of the material means that there is a risk that the junior psychiatrist will treat the psychotherapy patient in a different or special way. This in turn increases the risks of *boundary incursions*, and is another reason for good supervision of CBT practice.

Setting goals for the therapy and treatment plan

Part of the contract of therapy will be a setting of *therapy goals* that will have been agreed between the patient and therapist. There is no point agreeing vague, unreachable goals such as 'to be a better person' or to 'stop arguing with my partner'. They need to be:

- *realistic*
- *relevant* to the patient's presenting problems
- as *specific* as possible.

The specificity is to both allow a clear goal to work towards and be able to show when you have reached it. Therefore, to agree a goal: 'to go outdoors three times per day' may be realistic and may be relevant if the presenting complaint was inability to leave the home. It is possible to show when the goal has been achieved. Compare this goal to: 'go outdoors more'. It would not be clear at the end of therapy whether the goal had been achieved, or at least the extent to which it had been achieved.

It practice it is best not to make more than about three goals for therapy. The goals then help the therapist to construct a *treatment plan*. This is simply a map or outline of how the treatment will proceed. The following are potential goals and treatment plans for Sadie's therapy:

Sadie's agreed *goals* were:

1 to learn more about depression
2 to open all of my mail within two days of receiving it and always answer the phone
3 to feel good enough in my mood that I apply for and attend an evening course at Lanscombe College.

The agreed *treatment plan* was that treatment would progress in the following order (obviously reviewed depending on the outcome of each intervention):

1 to complete an activity diary
2 to complete activity-scheduling work, which will include a gradual increase in activities currently avoided (in particular contact with friends and answering the telephone)
3 an exposure hierarchy for opening the mail, followed by scheduling this activity into my week
4 reading the introduction to the practical problem-solving chapter in the *Overcoming Depression* book by Chris Williams
5 to learn about unhelpful thinking styles
6 to complete thought diaries
7 to complete risk-prevention work.

As any treatment can be conceptualised as having 'beginning', 'middle' and 'end' phases, it is useful to think of the tasks to be generally attempted during each of these phases. Generally these would be the following:

- *beginning*:
  - assessment, including initial 'baseline' rating scale scores
  - developing a provisional formulation

- setting agreed boundaries and contract of therapy (including 2–3 goals for therapy)
- working out a treatment plan
- development of therapeutic relationship
- instillation of hope
- *middle*
  - specific techniques to achieve specific targets of treatment
  - monitoring progress using clinical assessment and validated rating scales
  - extensive use of homework or practice tasks in between the sessions
  - review of formulation: is it still correct, are there new important elements to be included?
  - review of treatment: is it progressing reasonably? Are there problems, and if so how can they be addressed?
- *end*
  - relapse prevention work: how can the patient now plan for the future?
  - preparing for finishing the therapeutic contact (ending)
  - reviewing what went well, what didn't go well and what the patient has gained from CBT.

The structure of the session

The structure of 'the CBT session' has developed to make best use of time and to keep focused on the task at hand. However, the structure is for guidance and does not need to be slavishly stuck to at all costs. The standard structure for a CBT session flows in the following order:

- review of the *intervening week* (or other period since the previous session)
- setting the *agenda* of the session
- review of *previous session's homework task*
- main work or *focus* of the session
- *set homework*
- review the *session*.

Review of the intervening week

The events of the period since the past CBT session are discussed. This discussion will usually include significant changes in symptoms, life circumstances or treatments from other sources such as medication changes. If there have been significant events or changes then these can be added to the agenda for fuller discussion. The usual approach is to ask similar types of questions that you would in a standard clinical follow-up appointment.

Setting the agenda of the session

The patient and the therapist collaboratively need to set the agenda for the session. A question that would begin to decide upon the agenda could be: 'what specific issues would you want to work on this week to help you reach your goals?' Good agenda items help patients make progress on their treatment goals. If there are many issues and time is likely to be insufficient, then items will need to be prioritised and others will need to be worked on at home or carried over to another session. It is best to focus the session down to *one or two areas* only.

Review of the previous session's homework

As the majority of the work will be practised out of the session, it is always essential that the homework (or practice task) that was set in the previous session be reviewed. Nothing will stop your patient doing their homework quicker than failing to review their previous week's work!

Main work or focus of the session

The patient's treatment goals will have helped to define the specific tasks required for effective treatment. Keeping an overview of where the therapy is going is easier if these specific goals are kept in mind. The specific interventions will be some form of changing unhelpful thoughts and/or behaviours.

Set homework

This leads on from the session's interventions. Usually it will be to practise a skill tried out in the session, or a skill introduced earlier in treatment. This will help to *generalise* the changes made in therapy. Like any new skill, it needs practice to achieve competency. Homework also provides opportunities for *information gathering*, such as by using behavioural experiments or diaries of thoughts and behaviours to look for patterns that cannot always be predicted in the clinic.

Review of the session

Reflecting on the session by again asking what went well, what didn't go well, and what has been learnt is a strategy to achieve feedback and to review the content of the session. Asking whether the patient has been upset by anything discussed will help individuals who have difficulties with personal comments to practise voicing their thoughts and feelings. Finally, the *time and place* of the following appointment need to be agreed upon.

Structuring sessions when there is not much time

The traditional CBT hour-long (or often 50-minute) treatment session uses the above structure to maximise the effectiveness of the session by providing both a focus and structure for work. With a few modifications, the CBT session structure can be readily integrated into shorter clinical review sessions. To achieve this, clear choices need to be made regarding the focus and content of the session. In order to be realistic in terms of the time frame available, it may be necessary to focus on only one area in each session.

Supervision

There are three elements that need to be in place to enable the development of psychotherapy skills:

- *teaching*: being taught the therapy
- *clinical practice*: carrying out the therapy
- *supervision*: review of your therapy by someone else.

Why is supervision so important in psychotherapy?

Everyone engaged in delivering clinical interventions can benefit from clinical supervision. Supervision encourages reflection on the therapist's own thoughts and feelings, which may themselves interfere with good clinical judgement. We all have our blind spots and having someone to discuss issues with is essential. This is particularly important in psychotherapy because much of the therapeutic change is dependent upon general factors in the therapeutic relationship involving issues such as empathy, genuineness and rapport.

In supervision with trainees, the supervisor has additional roles. They have responsibilities for the patient and the trainee. The patient will know they are seeing someone in training but will expect to improve with treatment. The trainee is not expected to be especially skilled and so will need guidance. How does the supervisor provide this guidance? The most effective way is for the trainee to sit in or watch the supervisor doing therapy. The trainee can then see the process for himself or herself. Then they can start seeing patients and taping sessions either on video or audiotape, so that the supervisor can fulfil their joint responsibilities to patient and trainee. Recording all your sessions is good clinical practice, and with proper consent procedures, most patients agree to it.

What should you expect from supervision?

Supervision is an ideal situation to model and practice CBT interventions. This modelling can include cognitive and behavioural techniques, which can be *role-played* within the supervision session. The actual *format* of the supervision also tends to mimic that of a CBT treatment session. Therefore, good supervision will use time effectively and there will be a collaborative setting of the agenda. It will stick to the trainee's goals, review homework tasks and set new homework tasks for the following supervision session. Concentrating on one or two specific tasks per session will improve effectiveness. The goals of the training need to be clear. What do you what from this? What went well? What didn't go well? What did you learn? At the end of the training were your training goals met? You can expect your supervisor to help you try and reach your training goals, to be knowledgeable about the treatment and to be understanding of the difficulties of learning.

What should your supervisor expect from you?

Turning up prepared for supervision is a good start. The trainee also needs to have thought about items for the agenda and how they tie in to their learning objectives. Taping all of the therapy sessions and listening to them under supervision may feel uncomfortable but is a fast-track way of learning.

Emotional aspects of ending

Special care needs to be taken with finishing therapeutic contact. It needs to be discussed with the patient that this can be emotionally quite difficult. There are a number of potential reasons for this, including the fact that they may be used to their sessions – it may have in itself added structure to the week. They may have felt supported by the therapist and may have to some degree non-intentionally become *dependent on the contact*. This should be watched for throughout the therapy, and efforts made to reduce dependency. Nevertheless, even if the ending is spaced out over a number of weeks with less frequent sessions towards the end, some patients still find goodbyes difficult. In the authors' opinion this needs to be made explicit quite early on in treatment and normalised so that the patient does not deduce that they are abnormal for finding the ending of therapy difficult. The subject of ending therapy has traditionally been considered more in psychodynamic therapy because of the depth of the interpersonal relationship in that model. Nevertheless, the emotional aspect of ending therapy should still be considered and planned for when engaging in cognitive or behavioural therapies. The formulation should also indicate those patients who may have a problem here – such as those who easily *feel rejected* or who have formed very close dependent relationships with other people including professionals in the past. *Longer-term therapy* such as CBT for personality disorders is far more likely to induce emotional dependency issues. This is both because of the length of treatment and also because of the characteristics of the patient group. The preparation required for ending therapy – including an appreciation of the emotional impact that ending will have on the patient should be a routine part of the discussion within supervision.

MAIN POINTS

- Goal setting involves setting goals for the short, medium and the long term.
- A number of patient factors are likely to influence therapy, and therefore influence which patients are likely to be offered CBT. Generally patients with more chronic disorders, with co-existing diagnoses, more social problems, less motivation and who are less psychologically minded are the most difficult to treat.
- The CBT assessment involves more than taking a history. It is likely to incorporate formal questionnaires. It will also involve the creation of a formulation, an assessment of the patient's capacity to use the cognitive behavioural model, and an agreed treatment plan based on the goals of treatment.
- Completing validated questionnaires has a number of functions such as measuring progress of therapy over time and 'benchmarking' different services.
- Themes of the cognitive behavioural history include modulating, maintaining and protective factors.
- The five-areas formulation separates a situation and patient responses into its five constituent parts. The relationships between these five areas can then be explored.
- A 'linear' CBT formulation (based on the Beck *et al*, 1979 model of depression) shows how early life experiences shape schemas which can then become activated in later life to generate negative automatic thoughts (NATs). NATs then play a role in maintaining depression (as well as other conditions).
- This general 'linear' structure can be used to formulate other problem situations in addition to depression. It is also useful to formulate cases in some examinations.

- Each CBT session should be structured to include a review of the previous session, a review of the set homework from the previous session, agenda setting, the agreed work of the current session, and the setting of new homework for the period before the next session.
- Supervision of practice is important in CBT to prevent 'blind spots' of practice.
- The management of the ending of therapy with the patient is an important part of CBT practice as it is in other models of psychotherapy.

Further reading

- Beck AT, Rush AJ, Shaw BF and Emery G (1979) *Cognitive Therapy of Depression*. New York: Guilford Press.
- Moorey S (1996) Cognitive behaviour therapy for whom? *Advances in Psychiatric Treatment* **2**: 17–23.
- Williams C (2001) *Overcoming Depression: a five areas approach*. London: Arnold.

Chapter 6

General cognitive and behavioural techniques

Introduction • Common factors • Cognitive techniques • Behavioural techniques

Introduction

The primacy of thoughts and behaviours in the development and maintenance of symptoms of mental ill-health is the key component of the CBT model.

The aim of CBT is therefore to teach people to:

- identify their thoughts, behaviours, feelings, life situations, and physical systems
- evaluate how helpful they are
- consider and adopt alternative thoughts and behaviours.

How does a CBT therapist help their patients with this learning? We can categorise the active ingredients of therapy into:

- common factors
- cognitive techniques
- behavioural techniques.

Common factors

When we think about CBT we may initially think about the specific techniques that are part of the therapy. However, there are common factors present in most psychotherapies that lead to improvement in the patient's state. In fact some investigators argue that there is greater evidence for the efficacy of common factors than there is for specific treatments (Wampold and Messer, 2002).

So what are these common factors, and can we learn them? These common factors can be thought of as:

- the relationship between the patient and the therapist
- the personal attributes of the therapist.

The relationship between the patient and the therapist

The quality of this relationship has a proven association with outcome. How a patient gets on with their therapist is as complex as any human-to-human relationship. Some pairings just don't work. The ability to recognise this and do something about it is vital. When there are problems in the relationship between the patient and therapist then this needs to be worked upon (*see* Safran and Segal, 1990). Difficulties in the therapeutic relationship can even point to patterns of communication in the patient's life that may have created the presenting problems (a major emphasis of the work within psychodynamic psychotherapy). Identifying and practising new relating patterns can then be an essential part of therapy. In this way, patient–therapist relationship problems are an opportunity to learn. However, there are occasions when the breakdown in the relationship between patient and therapist is so severe that a change in therapist is the best option. Although this change obviously needs to be handled carefully, it can be an effective strategy.

The personal attributes of the therapist

Being *empathic, genuine,* and *holding unconditional positive regard* towards the patient are the attributes associated with the most effective therapists (Rogers, 1951). Being aloof, judgmental and acting as an expert are not. Relationships that are judged by the patient as *supportive* or *collaborative* likewise predict improved outcomes (Horvarth and Greenberg, 1989). Importantly, the quality of the therapeutic relationship as judged by the patient predicts outcome better than that judged by the therapist (Burns and Auerbach, 1996) – showing that as therapists we can sometimes misjudge how good our professional relationships are with our clients. There are *rating scales* that assess interpersonal effectiveness, and these can be effective tools to be used in supervision when listening to or watching session-tapes (e.g. the CTS-R: Newcastle CBT Centre and University of Newcastle Upon Tyne, 1999). The CTS-R places an overall rating on the effectiveness of a session of CBT. It incorporates a number of scales that are subjectively marked by the assessor who rates the therapy usually by observing a video- or audio-taped session (or less commonly by actually sitting in on the session itself). Some of these scales are predictable – such as the skill of introducing a cognitive or behavioural technique. Others are far more subjective and relate to the interpersonal relationship between the client and therapist. For example, one item measures the therapist's 'charisma' in his or her interaction with the client.

Although it is generally acknowledged that the therapeutic relationship is important for outcome, it is not yet clear why. Some have suggested that a good relationship works by *instilling hope*, others suggest that it encourages the client to complete in-session and homework tasks (i.e. it *allows the technical aspects* of CBT to continue unimpeded), while others have emphasised the importance of *modelling a positive relationship* that can be generalised to other relationships outside of therapy (*see* Waddington, 2002 for a review). Suggestions for maximising the potential of the therapeutic relationship are outlined below (headings from Waddington, 2002).

1   *Elicit the client's view of the therapeutic relationship*: note the findings of Burns and Auerbach, 1996 (above).

2 *Aim to generate hope via the therapeutic relationship.*
3 *Use cognitive skills to establish a good therapeutic relationship.* This may include the use of a clear formulation showing that the therapist understands the patient's situation (Persons, 1989).
4 *Attend to ruptures in the therapeutic relationship.*
5 *Aim for positive therapist characteristics.* This can be encouraged by close supervision and even therapy for the therapist (Bennett-Levy *et al*, 2004).
6 *Attend to generalisation from the therapeutic relationship.* This refers to the process whereby the client learns new, more helpful, ways of relating to others within therapy and then practises these in their relationships outside of therapy (Blackburn and Twaddle, 1996).
7 *Consider individual client issues in the therapeutic relationship.* This will be important, for example, when treating patients with issues relating to sensitivity to perceived rejection.
8 *Use supervision to monitor therapists' relationship skills* (e.g. by using the CTS-R).

Cognitive techniques

- Cognitive behavioural assessment
- Goal setting
- Practical problem solving
- Self-monitoring
- Cognitive restructuring (including use of thought diaries)
- Behavioural experiments

In the previous chapter we looked at *cognitive behavioural assessment, goal setting* and practical *problem-solving techniques.* We will discuss the other techniques in this chapter.

Self-monitoring (diary work)

Being competent in monitoring 'events' is arguably one of the most (if not *the* most important) skill in CBT. By 'events' we could be referring to almost any area in the 'five-areas model' (Williams, 2001). It could therefore be referring to 'behaviour' such as the number of times we brush our teeth, or wash our hands. It could be referring to something in the environment around us, such as the times that we are visited by friends or the times we are complimented by colleagues. Our mood and emotions can similarly be measured (albeit subjectively) as can the frequency and intensity with which we think certain thoughts. Often we don't just need to note whether something has happened or not, but the *degree* to which it has happened. Sometimes this is easy – so the number of times friends visit in the week can simply be recorded as '*discrete variables*'. However, when it comes to the degree that we believe a thought or the degree to which we feel low or angry we are dealing with '*continuous variables*'. We have to assign a figure – usually in percentage terms or as a figure 'out of ten', to describe the degree to which we are experiencing that thought or emotion.

The figure that we assign to a continuous variable is arbitrary – one person may be feeling 'a bit down' and describe themselves as 75% depressed, someone else

Table 6.1 Diary designed to monitor agitation and morning mood state

	Mon	Tues	Weds	Thurs
Time awoke finally in the morning				
Number of hours' sleep				
Mood in first hour after waking (0–100%, where higher score is better mood)				
Agitation level (0–10, where 10 is most agitation)				
What I did in the first hour – including what I ate/drank				
Took diazepam (yes/no)				

might describe the same subjective feeling as 40%. It doesn't matter that people differ – what is important is that the person filling in the diary sticks to their own way in which they rate. This is because we want to be able to compare rating scores between different situations and over different times. Therefore, it might be useful to know that a patient feels 40% agitated after 8 pm but 80–90% agitated at 5–6 am, and that this is a pattern that continues throughout the week. In this example, it may well indicate significant diurnal mood variation with associated symptoms of agitation. Being able to measure and explain this to the patient might be helpful to increase understanding and monitor response to treatment more accurately.

This principle of self-monitoring and keeping a structured diary can be extremely useful, not just in formal CBT, but also in most areas of psychiatry. For example, Table 6.1 shows a 'diary' designed by a junior psychiatrist to measure the degree of agitation and mood state in the mornings. It doesn't matter what you call this diary – mood diary, sleep diary, etc. What is important is the following:

- that the professional and the patient are both clear about *what they are measuring* and *how they are measuring it*. So, they agree in this example that agitation is a: 'feeling inside the chest of being wounded' (patient's description), and that higher scores out of ten equate to higher levels of agitation. This is important when measuring mood – one patient may prefer to describe 'levels of depression' out of ten, another by assigning a percentage where higher scores relate not to higher levels of depression but 'better mood', and so lower levels of depression. To a large extent it doesn't matter how the rating is scored so long as the system is kept to and is understood fully
- that the diary is *measuring all the variables* that are needed. In the above case it was important to measure what was eaten and drunk in those early hours. It turned out that the patient had been drinking diet cola containing caffeine, which aggravated the agitation

- that the person completing the diary completes it as *contemporaneously as possible* to the time period that it is referring to. The danger with filling in the above diary at the end of the week would be that details would be forgotten and mistakes made
- that the professional and patient look at the diary carefully after its completion. *Patterns are what are important.* Is there a pattern here between the intake of diazepam and the level of agitation, the level of agitation and the time that the patient wakes, and a pattern between the behaviour of the patient and the mood state? If the aim of the diary is to look for the effect of an intervention – such as the initiation of an antidepressant medication – then it is important to repeat the same diary with identical measures before and after the intervention has been started – remember the 'audit cycle'
- to complete the diary for an *adequate time scale*. Often patterns may not emerge until the diary has been completed for a number of weeks
- to be aware that *monitoring can change the behaviours* that are being measured without introducing any other interventions. Therefore, monitoring alcohol intake can reduce the person's intake. As the patient becomes aware of the extent of their behaviour it makes sense that they will try and change it. Some will be embarrassed and change their behaviour for the sake of the assessment – others will simply lie!

The monitoring of thoughts is even more difficult for many patients. This is probably because we are generally not accustomed to thinking about our thoughts – they pop into our heads and we generally accept what they are 'saying'. We need to practise noticing what our thoughts are telling us, the degree to which we believe them, and the effect that they have on our mood/ emotions, on our behaviour, and on physical feelings and symptoms (back to the five-areas model again (p. 70)!)

Cognitive restructuring

Task: spend a few moments thinking about your thinking

Imagine you believed the following thoughts as if they were 100% true:

- 'I am going to fail the exam'
- 'My partner is seeing someone else'
- 'I have to succeed for someone to love me'
- 'There's no future for me'

Pick one and think about the impact of that unhelpful thought on how you feel and what you would do. If you believed the thought, how would it affect your relationships, your views of the future and your thoughts about yourself?

Guided discovery

The above examples remind us of the impact of unhelpful thoughts, core beliefs and assumptions. Being able to identify these thoughts/feelings/behaviours is a

Table 6.2 Attempt to find other explanations for negative thoughts

Situation	Negative thoughts	Other explanations
Getting critical feedback for an essay	I am stupid	I didn't have much time to do this essay – the workload has been very heavy recently. I chose to do other things as well. The work is supposed to be challenging. Constructive criticism helps me to improve.
My partner does not want to see me tonight.	They don't care about me any more	They said they had to work tonight – this is probably true. We saw each other at the weekend and had a good time. He said some nice things to me lately and seemed caring the last time we met.

core skill of CBT. The therapist asks questions to understand the patient's view of things, not to simply change the patient's mind. Guided discovery is a style of asking questions that both gathers information and helps the patient to look at this information in different ways. For example, the therapist may ask what it was about the situation that was distressing, whether their coping strategy worked, whether they had ever used alternative strategies in the past, and whether this situation might have been addressed in any other ways. This information might otherwise have been difficult for the patient to access – it may lie outside of current awareness. The overall aim is to help the patient to *practise being able to view situations from different perspectives*. There is rarely just one way of thinking about a situation. There are usually several differing points of view. This general attitude of standing back from thoughts and seeing them as just one potential view of reality is extremely important within CBT and is referred to as the ability to '*decentre*'. Table 6.2 gives two examples of the process.

When our patients experience situations that they find very upsetting, many have difficulty balancing their immediate unhelpful thoughts with alternative views. This ability to think about a situation in a variety of ways is an important step in the process of gathering information to challenge unhelpful thoughts. Much of this work will rely on the patient completing specially designed forms, which they complete when upset. Filling in such a *thought diary* helps to capture unhelpful thoughts and the impact of these thoughts on other 'areas' (of the five-areas model). The easiest way to teach patients how to use thought diaries is to introduce them inside the session. It is best to illustrate their use using a simple example from the patient's life.

Completing a thought diary

Different versions of thought diaries have similar layouts, but can differ to a degree. For example, some authors ask the client to identify the type of cognitive distortion shown in their thought as well as the actual thought itself (e.g. Williams, 2001). Other thought diaries simply get the patient to identify and then challenge the content of the thought without identifying the type of cognitive distortion (e.g. Greenberger and Padesky, 1995). Thought diaries are particularly useful in circumstances when the patient notices a change for the worse in their emotional state – perhaps when they suddenly feel low or angry. It is very often the case that an unhelpful or biased thought lies behind the change so that the patient can practice identifying and then challenging these thoughts in order to prevent worsening of these negative emotional states. At least to start with, it is important that the patient *writes down* the content of thought records rather than trying to 'work it out' in their head. This is to remain focused and to allow the patient to simultaneously examine large amounts of 'evidence' in order to arrive at a balanced conclusion regarding the validity of the distressing thought. The following steps are used in most thought diaries, but the terms used here are from Greenberger and Padesky, 1995. (An example of a patient's responses, a secretary called 'Helen', is written in italics.)

1 The circumstances (of the emotional change)

- *'10:30 am, at work, about to go into the administrator's office to ask for annual leave to which I am entitled, but which is more than some of my colleagues are taking.'*

2 The emotions experienced at the time and the extent to which those emotions are experienced

It is important to rate these emotions using an agreed scale – the scales most commonly used are percentages although other scales such as colours or marks out of 10 can also be used.

- *Shame at 80%*
- *Fear at 60%*
- *Sadness at 30%*

3 The automatic thoughts experienced at the time

The thought most closely associated with the emotion (sometimes called the 'hot thought' – Greenberger and Padesky, 1995) then needs to be chosen with a rating of the degree to which that thought is believed. Again, as in 2, any scale can be used, in practice most use percentages).

- *'She will sneer at me.'*
- *'I will not know what to say and will make a fool of myself.'*
- *'My colleagues all think that I'm ineffective.'*
- *'She's going to make a fuss.'*
- The most prominent thought (the 'hot thought') and the one linked most closely with the feeling of shame: *'My colleagues all think that I'm ineffective': the degree to which I believe this = 90%.*

4 Evidence supporting the 'hot thought'

Here all the evidence that supports the 'hot thought' is listed.

- *'The administrator sent me an unpleasant e-mail last year about staff taking excessive annual leave.'*
- *'The administrator always seems to sneer at me and rarely makes eye contact.'*
- *'I've been off work with depression for four months and that has been hard on the department.'*
- *'I often think of myself as being ineffective.'*
- *'I presented a poor report 3 weeks ago.'*

- *'Jim my boss said in my annual review that I needed to improve upon my ''organisational skills''.'*

5 Evidence not supporting the 'hot thought'

Here the patient is encouraged to write down as much evidence as they can muster that goes against their 'hot thought'.

- *'The administrator sneers at everyone!'*
- *'She is very unpopular in the department – Debbie confirmed this when we spoke over lunch.'*
- *'I am well liked and I got lots of well wishes when I was unwell.'*
- *'I have presented much better reports in the past.'*
- *'People often come to me for advice.'*
- *'I have been told by a few people that my ''people skills'' are good – and if there are presentations to be made to the public they seem to ask me to do them.'*
- *'I am just back from depression and 4 months off – it would take a while for anyone to get back into ''the swing of things'' – I think that's also why the report was difficult for me.'*
- *'Just because I think of myself as ineffective it doesn't really mean I am – as my friend Sophie said, I am my own worst critic.'*
- *'Nobody has actually said to me ever that my general work is poor or that I am ineffective.'*

6 The 'balanced conclusion' and the degree to which it is believed

The degree to which the initial 'hot thought' is now believed is also re-rated

The balanced conclusion is the new belief drawn from all of the evidence listed in points 4 and 5 above. It may be completely different from the original 'hot thought' or it may be an altered, more balanced, version of that initial thought. The degree to which this new balanced conclusion is believed is rated.

- *'I've been off ill for some time and am managing well in the circumstances. My organisational skills are not my strong point – but I am good with people and that's OK. Really there is no proof that everyone thinks I'm ineffective – maybe a bit disorganised but everyone has their weak and strong points.'*
- *The degree to which I believe this new 'balanced thought' = 85%.'*
- The client now goes back to re-rate how much they now believe the initial 'hot thought' that they noted down in point no. 3 above.
- *'The degree to which I now believe the ''hot thought'': ''My colleagues all think that I'm ineffective'' = 50%.'*

7 Re-rate the emotions (as previously noted in point 2 above)

- *Shame at 30%*
- *Fear at 40%*
- *Sadness at 10%*

In this example, therefore, the extent to which the patient believed the original thought was reduced and the new balanced conclusion was judged to be accurate. The effect on the patient's emotions was positive (a reduction in negative emotions including sadness).

Tables 6.3 and 6.4 illustrate this general process of identifying and then challenging biased and unhelpful thoughts. The author (Williams, 2001) separates

Table 6.3 Thought investigation worksheet (from *Overcoming Depression: a five areas approach* © Dr CJ Williams (2001) Reproduced with permission of Edward Arnold (Publishers) Ltd)

1 Situation/relationship or practical problem when your mood altered	2 Altered emotional and physical feelings	3 What immediate thoughts are present at the time?	4 What unhelpful thinking style(s) occur?	5 Impact of the immediate thought(s)
Think in detail: where am I, what am I doing? Consider: • *the time*: what time of day is it? • *the place*: where am I? • *the people*: who is present, who am I with? • *the events*: what has been said/what events happened?	Am I: • low or sad? guilty? • worried, tense, anxious or panicky? • angry or irritable? • ashamed? a State the feelings clearly. Try to be as precise as possible. If more than one feeling occurs, underline the most powerful feeling. b How powerful is this feeling? (0–100%) c Note down any strong physical sensations you notice	What is going through my mind? How do I see: • myself, how do others see me? • the current events/situation • what might happen in the future? • my own body, behaviour or performance? • any memories or images? a State the thought(s) clearly. Try to be as precise as possible. If more than one thought occurs, underline the most powerful thought b Rate how strongly you believe the most powerful thought at the time (0–100%)	1 Bias against myself 2 Putting a negative slant on things (negative mental filter) 3 Having a gloomy view of the future/jumping to the worst conclusion 4 Negative view about how others see me (mind-reading) 5 Bearing all responsibility 6 Making extreme statements/rules e.g. using *must, should, ought, always,* and *never* statements If any of the styles are present, you have identified an extreme thought	a What did I do differently? Consider any: • reduced or avoided activity • unhelpful behaviours b What was the impact on: • myself? • my view of others? • how I felt? • what I said? • what I did? Overall, was the impact helpful or unhelpful? If there is an unhelpful impact, you have identified an unhelpful thought
Situation	a My feelings b Powerfulness (0–100%) c Physical sensations	My immediate thought(s): a state the thoughts clearly If you have noticed more than one thought, underline the most powerful thought c Rate your belief in the most powerful thought at the time 0% 100% |- - - - - - - - - -|- - - - - - - - - -|	Which thinking styles are present? (please state numbers or types)	a What did I do differently? b Overall is it helpful or unhelpful for me to believe the thought?

Table 6.4 Thought challenge worksheet (from *Overcoming Depression: a five areas approach* © Dr CJ Williams (2001) Reproduced with permission of Edward Arnold (Publishers) Ltd)

6 Reasons supporting the immediate thought	7 Evidence against the immediate thought	8 Come to a balanced conclusion	9 My plan for putting the balanced conclusion into practice
List all the reasons why I believed the immediate thought at the time	• Is there anything to make me think the thought is incorrect? • Are there any other ways of explaining the situation that are more accurate? • If I wasn't feeling like this, what would I say? • Would I tell a friend who believed the same thought that they were wrong? • What would other people say? • Have I heard *different opinions* from others about the thought?	Use the answers from columns 6 and 7 to try to come up with a *balanced* and *helpful* conclusion. Look for a *balanced conclusion* that you can believe. This should be based on *all* the information you have available to you and bear in mind the reasons for and against believing the immediate thought	• How can I change what I do to reinforce my balanced conclusion? • How can I undermine my immediate negative thought by acting against it?
My evidence supporting the immediate thought (write in):	My evidence against the immediate thought (write in):	My balanced conclusion (write in): a Rating of my belief in the balanced thought: 0% 100% |– – – – – – – – – – –| b Re-rating of my belief in the immediate thought: 0% 100% |– – – – – – – – – – –|	My plan for putting the balanced conclusion into practice (write in):

the process into two worksheets – the 'thought investigation' worksheet and the 'thought challenge' worksheet. He tries to encourage the patient to consider the impact of the biased thoughts within the 'five-areas formulation', which has already been described in Chapter 5. Particularly useful steps are columns 5 and 9. These are often omitted from thought records, but are a useful means of encouraging the patient to think about the effects of their biased thoughts on their behaviour, and then to consider the potential impact of the new balanced thoughts on their future behaviour.

If our belief has changed then we need to push ourselves to behave differently in line with our new balanced belief. If we consider our example again from above – Helen – then column 4 would have been completed as:

What unhelpful thinking style(s) occur?

• *'Numbers 1 and 3: having a bias against myself and having a gloomy view of the future.'*

Column 5 would be completed as:

a What did I do differently?

• *'I have avoided sorting out my annual leave because I think the team will think I don't deserve it. This has stopped me from being able to plan my leave activities.'*
• *'I have also avoided putting myself forward for tasks within the team, such as audit projects.'*
• *'I have avoided Jim [the manager] in case he forwards me for tasks that I will fail at and be criticised about.'*

B Overall, is it helpful or unhelpful for me to believe the thought?

• *'Unhelpful.'*

Finally, column 9 would have been completed as:

My plan for putting the balanced conclusion into practice

• *'The main thing I need to do is to go ahead and meet with Kelly. When I do I will maintain eye contact instead of looking downwards as I normally do when I meet her.'*
• *'I shall try and meet with my manager (Jim) to see what has changed in the department and what opportunities there are for me (as opposed to general avoidance).'*
• *'I should put myself forward for more projects – as a start I shall elect to do the audit of customer contacts.'*

As you can see, all of the other columns within these two worksheets correspond to the general format of a *thought diary* – such as the one by Greenberger and Padesky (1995) outlined earlier in this chapter. These worksheets give suggestions or clues in the upper part, leaving the lower spaces for the patient to write their responses. By filling in this form when upset, and by slowing down and spending time thinking and asking questions of themselves, patients develop new insights into their problems. *It is important to note that it takes time and repeated practice for anybody to change their negative thinking habits.*

Behavioural experiments

Why do behavioural experiments?

All of us use behaviour to validate our thoughts, assumptions and beliefs. In anxiety disorders, safety behaviours reflect assumptions – if I do X then Y will happen. For example: 'if I let go of this shopping trolley I'll begin to shake and go out of control'. Discovering what patients predict will happen if they do not engage in safety behaviours, and then testing out what actually happens is a powerful challenge to these unhelpful assumptions.

Background theory

In the world of adult education the Lewin–Kolb Learning Circle (Lewin, 1946; Kolb, 1984; *see* Figure 6.1) is a theory that has become widespread when developing effective learning. The circle is made of four stages that should be repeatedly traversed for continued learning.

The Lewin–Kolb learning cycle can be used in any learning situation. The benefit of this approach is that when you reflect you can work on the three levels of unhelpful thinking (automatic thoughts, assumptions and core beliefs).

Being able to identify and challenge thoughts is useful but is removed from reality to some extent – by definition it's a task very much 'in your head'. The experiential is more real and often more convincing. So planning to do something that makes alternative thoughts more real, and unhelpful thoughts less convincing is *one of the most powerful ways of challenging unhelpful thoughts*. It can also be helpful to plan experiments where patients find identifying alternative thoughts very difficult.

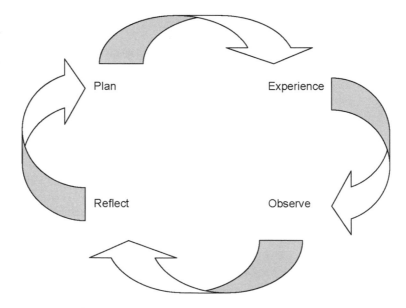

Figure 6.1 The Lewin–Kolb Learning Cycle (Lewin, 1946; Kobb, 1984) adapted from Bennett-Levy J, Butler G, Fennell M *et al.* (eds) (2004) *Oxford Guide to Behavioural Experiments in Cognitive Therapy*, with permission from Oxford University Press.

The types of experiments can therefore be:

- thought testing
- discovery
- activity based
- observational.

The thought-challenging worksheet will have identified:

1   the problem
2   the unhelpful thought associated with it
3   the percentage belief in this unhelpful thought
4   an alternative thought or thoughts
5   the percentage belief in this alternative thought or thoughts.

Now in the planning of the experiment we as the therapist are thinking of ways to reduce the belief in the identified unhelpful belief.

So the experiment could be to simply try out a new approach. Box 6.1 is an outline of the steps that can be used to structure behavioural experiments.

Box 6.1   Steps that can be used to structure behavioural experiments

(The headings are taken from Bennettt-Levy J, Butler G, Fennell M *et al.* (eds) (2004) *Oxford Guide to Behavioural Experiments in Cognitive Therapy*, with permission from Oxford University Press). The current authors have added the example.

- *Problem*: 'I have nothing to do this Friday night.'
- *Target cognition*: 'My friend hasn't phoned to ask me out because she doesn't like me much.' *Belief* = *85%*
- *Alternative perception*: 'If I phone her I can make an arrangement to meet on Friday. She will agree because she likes me.' *Belief* = *25%*
- *Prediction*: 'She will say she has already got something planned.'
- *Experiment*: 'I will phone my friend at 7 pm and suggest meeting on Friday night.'
- *Result*: 'I phoned my friend and she agreed to meet up on Friday.'
- *Reflection*: 'We talked on the phone for ages. I guess she was glad to hear from me after all.'
- *New rating*:
  - 'My friend hasn't phoned to ask me out because she doesn't like me much.' *Belief* = *10%*
  - 'If I phone her I can make an arrangement to meet on Friday. She will agree because she likes me.' *Belief* = *100%*
- *Further work*: 'Phone my friend and arrange to go out next week.'

It is important to try and observe thoughts and feelings before, during and after experiments. Note any changes in body sensations or physical symptoms. The patient can record how they are behaving and how they are relating to others. How are they responding to the environment? It is important to record the impact of the experiment on the target cognitions and/or target behaviours.

Reflect

What went well, what didn't go well, what have you learnt?

The ultimate goal is for the belief in the target cognition to reduce to 0%, and the belief in the alternative to rise to 100%. This measure of the extent of the belief change can help to answer the question: 'what would have to happen to bring the belief in the target cognition down to 0%?'

Further work may involve follow-on experiments. If possible think of ways to build on the initial experiment. This will help to reinforce the validity of the new thought and generalise the technique.

Encouraging patients to confront situations they have previously avoided involves a degree of risk-taking by the patient. The therapeutic relationship and an understanding of the specific goals of these behavioural experiments will help the patient to overcome this fear.

Repeated rehearsal and reinforcement may be required for many long-held unhelpful beliefs. The hope is that the patient will plan and independently carry out their own experiments.

Behavioural techniques

In traditional behaviour therapy there is an emphasis on changing behaviours rather than thoughts. If thoughts (cognitions) do change, they are considered to do so as a consequence of the changed behaviour. As already described, there has generally been a coming-together of cognitive and behavioural ideas, but listed below are some of the common techniques that can be thought of as originating in behaviour therapies:

- systematic desensitisation and graded exposure in vivo
- flooding
- exposure and response prevention
- relaxation therapy
- modelling
- behavioural chain analysis
- activity diary keeping and activity scheduling

Revision: conditioning (*see* Chapter 2)

- Behavioural techniques use the concepts of classical and operant conditioning.
- In operant conditioning reinforcement increases the probability that the person will repeat behavioural responses.
- In classical conditioning two or more stimuli become unconsciously

paired so that the person responds to the new conditioned stimulus as they did to the unconditioned stimulus.

- In practice (as in the example given below – enuresis alarms) there are elements of both types of conditioning in complex behaviour patterns. For example learning to associate the sensation of the full bladder with the bell (classical conditioning), and learning that setting the alarm off through urinating (behaviour) will lead to negative consequences (having to get out of bed) – operant conditioning.

Enuresis alarms are the most effective treatment of nocturnal enuresis. The bell and pad technique is an example of an enuresis alarm and is a form of behavioural therapy often used to treat nocturnal enuresis in children. A pad is placed underneath the bed sheets and connected to an alarm system that sounds every time that urine makes contact with a sensor. The aim is to train the child to learn to respond to a full bladder. More recent techniques include a sensor attached to the child's underwear, with the alarm connected to the wrist or pyjama collar, as many parents complained that the alarm wakes everyone in the house except the enuretic child. In these cases it is very important to ensure that the child is fully awake after the alarm goes off, otherwise the cycle of sensation and feedback is never completed.

Systematic desensitisation and graded exposure in vivo

The behavioural techniques of systematic desensitisation (SD) and graded exposure in vivo (GE) have been the mainstay of the treatment of phobias since the late 1950s.

Systematic desensitisation (SD) uses relaxation and exposure together, based on the premise that fear and relaxation states are incompatible. The patient is trained in relaxation techniques (*see* below). The patient and therapist then construct a hierarchy of anxiety-provoking situations. Then the patient is exposed to the items from the list, starting with the least anxiety-inducing items, in a graded way while inhibiting the anxiety by relaxation. This can be exposure in the imagination, by virtual reality or to the real feared situation.

More commonly nowadays, exposure is simply graded without the use of relaxation techniques. This is *graded exposure in vivo* (GE). The aim is to allow the patient to fully habituate to the anxiety-provoking situation without the use of relaxation techniques. It has been observed that patients may recruit relaxation as a 'safety behaviour'. For example, someone who experiences panic on exposure to a stimulus may try and manage the symptoms by relaxation techniques. While this may reduce the panic to a degree, it is unlikely to get rid of the symptoms completely, as the person never learns that the stimulus or the resulting panic symptoms are not truly threatening. GE is used for many problems such as panic, phobias and PTSD, and is discussed in more detail in the sections relating to these disorders.

Flooding

In common with SD and GE, flooding is another form of exposure. The aim of flooding remains the same – habituation. This technique is based on the exposure of the patient to the feared object or situation in a *non-graded* way, where escape from the situation is prevented, until the anxiety eventually diminishes. This can take over an hour and is obviously distressing. With adequate preparation, flooding is effective for some patients and some prefer this 'all or nothing' approach to a graded exposure regime. Flooding has to be carried out with care – there are many risks. The patient may be so overwhelmed that they remove themselves from the situation so that habituation does not occur. In contrast, they may now view the feared situation as even more overwhelming than they previously thought. Therefore, they become 'sensitised' to the situation, and the associated anxiety increases in strength. In the authors' experience most patients prefer, and are better suited towards, graded exposure in vivo.

Exposure and response prevention

This behavioural treatment is perhaps best known as the major approach used in patents with OCD. It does, however, have other applications, such as in the treatment of bulimia and overeating, substance misuse and gambling. It consists of graded exposure to situations that are known to provoke obsessional thoughts or impulses – such as the impulse to eat or gamble some money. The patient then implements self-imposed prevention of the compulsive act. By doing this gradually and with repeated exposures, the patient's anxiety on exposure to the stimulus subsides, and their urge to carry out the compulsive act will also subside over time. In common with other exposure regimes, the patient must also refrain from avoidance or safety behaviours. *See* Chapters 11 and 13 on OCD and bulimia nervosa for more information.

Relaxation therapy

Relaxation therapy may take place in groups or in one-to-one sessions with the therapist. Most relaxation techniques train the patient to relax muscles by using cycles of contraction and relaxation. Initially, each muscle group is relaxed individually. Later, the patient may become able to rapidly relax muscles throughout the body. It has non-specific value in many psychological states, and more specifically in anxiety disorders. Although many therapists use relaxation therapy from time to time, its position within CBT is debated. It is important that the patient does not recruit the relaxation techniques as further 'safety behaviours'. Relaxation techniques can be useful to actually get the patient in a position to allow exposure to occur in the first place, where anxiety levels have risen so high that the exposure is at risk of sensitising the patient rather than encouraging habituation.

Modelling

Used within the therapeutic context, modelling refers to the process where the therapist first carries out the action that is feared/avoided by the patient. The patient observes this and then attempts to carry out the behaviour in question him or herself. The underlying theory is of *social learning*. An example where modelling is frequently used is in the treatment of simple phobias. The therapist may model the safety of spiders by first touching the spider or allowing the spider onto themselves, before the patient attempts to expose him or herself to the same. Modelling requires patient identification with the model.

Behavioural chain analysis

Behavioural chain analysis is based on the observation that behaviour is maintained by reinforcing consequences. If the consequences are altered, then the problematic behaviours will also change. The approach works with a large variety of problems, both psychiatric and non-psychiatric.

An example of this might be a child who habitually climbs into bed with his parents. Behaviour modification is based on identifying the reinforcing consequences (e.g. the attention from the parents) and then modifying them. Thus, the parents might be instructed to return the child to bed with a standardised clear message each time he tries to get into bed with them. At first there is an extinction burst, that is an increase in the undesired behaviour, before the behaviour decreases and eventually stops altogether.

For any problem behaviour (e.g. comfort eating, deliberate self-harm, and aggressive behaviours), a behavioural chain analysis can be created. This will help to identify the activities that reinforce the behaviour.

Activity diary keeping and activity scheduling

Keeping a diary of one's activities through the day is a mainstay technique within CBT. Although the exact detail of the information gathered varies, most activity diaries record the principal activity carried out within a set period (usually hourly). In addition, they usually record whether the activity carried out gives the patient a sense of pleasure and also a sense of achievement (sometimes termed 'mastery'). Table 6.5 is an example of how an activity diary may look once completed. It is based upon a man in his early 40s with depression. The diary was completed over 3 weeks (only 3 days are shown in Table 6.5). Here, the diary uses 2-hour time periods because the patient found it difficult to remember to complete the diary each hour.

The following were the conclusions drawn by therapist and patient from the diary in Table 6.5.

- ruminating is a really powerful way of making my mood drop – this shocked me
- if I start to ruminate in the morning my mood stays low all day!
- staying in bed in the morning past 8–9 am makes my mood worse
- going back to bed makes my mood worse
- meeting with friends – e.g. Jeff, Sandy – makes me feel better
- activities that give a sense of achievement such as making dinner, or even shopping, which I hate, make me feel better in my mood
- even little things such as getting something from the corner shop can make me feel some achievement
- having my morning routine of paper and coffee helps keep my mood up.

Table 6.5 'My activity diary' (only 3 days of week's diary shown)

	Mon	Tues	Weds
5–7 am	Mood = 2 Lay in bed Ach = 0 Pl = 0	Mood = 1 Pacing around room Ach = 0 Pl = 0	Mood = 2 Lay in bed Ach = 0 Pl = 2
7–9 am	Mood = 4 Got ready Ach = 5 Pl = 3	Mood = 1 Tea, sitting in living room Ach = 0 Pl = 3	Mood = 3 Lay in bed Ach = 0 Pl = 2
9–11 am	Mood = 5 Walked to corner shop Ach = 6 Pl = 2	Mood = 4 Walked to town Ach = 0 Pl = 0	Mood = 2 Lay in bed ruminating Ach = 0 Pl = 1
11 am–1 pm	Mood = 3 Watched TV Ach = 0 Pl = 2	Mood = 4 Had coffee, read paper Ach = 1 Pl = 5	Mood = 1 Lay in bed ruminating Ach = 0 Pl = 0
1–3 pm	Mood = 6 Met Sandy for coffee Ach = 6 Pl = 7	Mood = 5 Got shopping in Ach = 6 Pl = 1	Mood = 2 Watched TV Ach = 0 Pl = 1
3–5 pm	Mood = 5 Went to video shop alone Ach = 5 Pl = 3	Mood = 6 Picked up Jeff from work Ach = 5 Pl = 6	Mood = 0 Back to bed ruminating Ach = 0 Pl = 0
5–7 pm	Mood = 6 Watched video alone Ach = 2 Pl = 6	Mood = 6 Had dinner with Jeff Ach = 7 Pl = 6	Mood = 3 Got up, made dinner Ach = 6 Pl = 4
7–9 pm	Mood = 3 Sitting thinking about me Ach = 0 Pl = 0	Mood = 7 Dennis and Jeff around Ach = 6 Pl = 7	Mood = 2 Watched TV ruminated Ach = 0 Pl = 0
9–11 pm	Mood = 4 Made then ate meal Ach = 5 Pl = 4	Mood = 7 Watched TV Ach = 3 Pl = 5	Mood = 1 Lay in bed Ach = 0 Pl = 0
11 pm–1 am	Mood = 5 Watched TV – then bed at 1 am Ach = 5 Pl = 5	Mood = 4 TV in bed then sleep ?time Ach = 3 Pl = 4	Mood = 1 Lay in bed Ach = 0 Pl = 0
1–3 am	Mood = 3 Awake but OK Ach = 0 Pl = 3	Sleep	Mood = 1 Lay in bed sleep ?time Ach = 0 Pl = 0

As soon as possible after each time period the patient notes down the principal activity carried out, a rating of mood (mood = rate out of 10 where higher is better mood), the degree of pleasure (Pl = rate out of 10 where higher is more pleasure), and degree of achievement or mastery from the activity (Ach = rate out of 10 where higher is a greater sense of achievement).

As outlined already, simply keeping a diary can change activity levels, probably because the patient's attention is focused on the subject. Monitoring activity helps to identify patterns of activity and the impact of these patterns on mood. Probably the most common pattern is a reduction of total activities, but a particular reduction in those activities that previously would have given the patient a sense of pleasure or achievement is also seen. This very often includes activities such as sport, exercise and socialising – all activities that help to maintain our moods and give a sense of pleasure and meaning. Alternatively patients may have diaries full of activities but have little time for themselves to schedule in pleasure pursuits. Other diaries are lacking in activities that give a sense of achievement or mastery, but do still contain pleasurable activities.

Once the patterns in the diary have been identified the next stage may be to complete an *activity schedule*. One of the fundamentals of cognitive behavioural therapy for depression involves the therapist and client working together to schedule activities that are going to be completed, usually in the week ahead. By increasing pleasurable and/or activities that give a sense of achievement, the aim is to improve mood. Some patients need to schedule in fewer total activities – but more of a certain type, perhaps those that give a sense of pleasure. In general, patients need a balance between pleasurable and achievement activities – normally about half of each type. The activity schedule may be completed on a similar diary sheet to the activity diary (but it obviously now applies prospectively). Table 6.6 shows 4 days of an activity schedule that may have been completed based on the findings of the diary in Table 6.5. Not every hour needs to be completed as long as there are enough activities of the right type scheduled in through the week. Here

Table 6.6 'My activity schedule' (only 4 days shown of week's schedule) Remember – ruminating makes my mood drop!

	Mon	*Tues*	*Weds*	*Thurs*
7–9 am	Get up before 9 am	Get up before 9 am	Get up before 9 am	Get up before 9 am
9–11 am				To Tamworth skiing till 7–8 pm!!
11 am–1 pm	Lunch with Sam in town	Paper and coffee	Paper and coffee	
1–3 pm	Ask Sam if she wants to go to gallery – if not go alone			
3–5 pm	Gallery	Pick up Jeff from work		
5–7 pm	Make dinner	Dinner with Jeff	Make dinner	
7–9 pm	'Sci-fi night' with James	Dennis and Jeff around	Do tax return	
9–11 pm	Home after James' house		Do tax return	Ask Jeff etc if they want to come in when we get back
11 pm–1 am	Aim for bed before 12	Aim for bed before 12	Aim for bed before 12	Aim for bed before 12

the patient has reminded himself about the effect of ruminating at the top of the schedule. The sheet needs to be kept safe, and preferably visible to remind the patient of the tasks to be attempted through the week. This patient pinned his schedule on his refrigerator!

MAIN POINTS

- The active ingredients of CBT can be categorised as common factors, cognitive techniques and behavioural techniques.
- The common factors are the therapeutic relationship factors and personal attributes of the therapist.
- Effective therapists (not just in CBT!) are genuine, empathic and hold unconditional positive regard (Rogers, 1951).
- Suggested ways of improving the therapeutic relationship include: eliciting the patient's view of the relationship and using supervision to monitor the therapist's relationships.
- Diaries aim to identify patterns in the same variable over time and relationships between different variables.
- Diaries need to be carefully designed so that it is clear what they measure and how they are measuring it. They also need to be completed over an adequate time scale so that patterns can emerge, and as contemporaneously to the events as possible.
- Cognitive restructuring can be achieved by many means including thought diaries, guided discovery and the completion of behavioural experiments.
- Thought records test out the accuracy of a thought by listing all the evidence that both supports and refutes it.
- Behavioural experiments test out the accuracy of thoughts and beliefs and then test out the accuracy of other alternative beliefs. It is important to plan follow-up experiments to help to reinforce the belief in these new alternative ways of viewing a situation.
- Systematic desensitisation, graded exposure in vivo, flooding and exposure and response prevention are all forms of exposure, and therefore, all have the underlying aim of habituation.
- Completing activity diaries and activity schedules are key interventions used in depression. The aim of activity scheduling is to help to balance (and usually increase) the daily frequency of behaviours that give either a sense of pleasure or a sense of mastery (achievement).

Further reading

- Bennett-Levy J, Butler G, Fennel M *et al.* (eds) (2004) *Oxford Guide to Behavioural Experiments in Cognitive Therapy*. Oxford: Oxford University Press.
- Greenberger D and Padesky C (1995) *Mind Over Mood: change how you feel by changing the way you think*. London: The Guilford Press.
- Williams C (2001) *Overcoming Depression: a five areas approach*. London: Arnold.

Part 3

Cognitive behavioural therapy applied to specific disorders

Chapter 7

Cognitive behavioural therapy applied to depression

The models • Assessment and formulation • The treatment

The models

Most cognitive behavioural formulations of depression are based on the original cognitive model of depression developed by Aaron T. Beck (see Beck *et al*, 1979). Beck used three main concepts within his model: the negative cognitive triad of depression, cognitive errors and the concept of the schema. The *cognitive triad of depression refers* to the depressed individual's tendency to view themselves, the world and the future, in a predominantly negative manner. These three areas are often portrayed as a triangle with the self, world, and the future at each corner. Evidence of this negative cognitive triad of depression is frequently heard in conversations with people who are depressed: 'I'm totally useless', 'You're no longer safe nowadays, I've stopped going out' and: 'I can't see a future any more, everything's grey'. *Cognitive errors* (also described as 'cognitive distortions' or 'faulty information processing') are characteristic errors in the process of thinking that help to maintain the negative beliefs that make up the cognitive triad. They were listed in Table 2.2.

Chris Williams has tried to simplify Beck's cognitive model of depression and uses different terms to describe the above cognitive errors (*see* Table 7.1).

As can be seen from Table 7.1, Williams' list of unhelpful thinking styles does not completely map onto Beck's cognitive errors. Some, such as 'having a bias against yourself' relate also to the negative cognitive triad of having a negative view of the self.

Beck's final concept within his cognitive model of depression was that of the '*schema*'. Many people also refer to schemas as 'core beliefs'. In essence, schemas can be seen as deeply held beliefs that have their origins primarily in childhood, and which form the lenses through which events and experiences are interpreted. Therefore, if someone has a schema: 'I am vulnerable', then a request to give a presentation to colleagues may be viewed very differently from someone who has a schema: 'I am special'. Beck hypothesised that in depression 'latent' negative schemas that have been formed in childhood become *activated* by a *precipitating event*. Once a schema is activated it: 'is the basis for molding data into cognitions . . . He categorizes and evaluates his experiences through the matrix of schemas' (Beck

Table 7.1 Chris Williams' 'Unhelpful thinking styles' (Headings taken from *Overcoming Depression: a five areas approach* © Dr CJ Williams (2001) Reproduced with permission of Edward Arnold (Publishers) Ltd.)

Unhelpful thinking style and example	Description of thinking style
1 A bias against yourself: 'I'm just hopeless – she'll get the job, I don't have a chance'	Williams also describes this as 'being your own worst critic'.
2 Putting a negative slant on things: 'The exam was awful – of the 180 questions I know I got five wrong!'	This refers to the tendency to downplay the positive aspect of a situation and talk-up the negative aspects of it. Williams also describes this as having a 'negative mental filter'.
3 Having a gloomy view of the future: 'If I ever go into debt I just know I'll never get out of it again'	Often called 'catastrophising', this refers to the tendency to imagine the worst happening, despite a lack of evidence that it will.
4 A negative view of how others see you: 'She thinks I look unattractive – I just know it – there's no point in ever saying hello'	This is the tendency to jump to negative conclusions about the way other people see you, based on inaccurate or inadequate information.
5 Bearing all responsibility: 'If anything goes wrong while I'm manager today I know I'll lose my job'	Similar to Beck's 'personalising', this is the tendency to take undue responsibility for people or situations.
6 Making extreme statements or rules: 'We have an awful relationship – we do nothing but argue!'	This equates to Beck's 'absolutistic thinking'.

et al, 1979, pp. 12–13). The development of negative schemas relates to the experiences and relationships that a child forms. As such it closely links with Bowlby's attachment theory (*see* Scher *et al*, 2004). This development of schemas and assumptions that predispose the person to having negative automatic thoughts (NAT's) is shown in Figure 2.3. It is important to know this 'linear' model well, as it forms the basis of many simple cognitive behavioural formulations.

Other models in addition to those of Beck have shaped the CBT approach to depression. Probably the most influential are those relating to activity levels and behavioural change. Lewinsohn *et al* (1986) suggest that depression is the result of repetitive and non-rewarding lifestyles. This model is linked with the use of *activity scheduling* and *behavioural activation* in CBT for depression. The general aims are to increase activity in general (including exercise), but also specifically to increase those stimulating and *pleasurable* activities that give a sense of *reward and achievement*. Activity diaries and scheduling are described further in Chapter 6. Another influential model has been that of depression as a condition maintained by *poor problem-solving skills* (D'Zurilla, 1986). This model has encouraged the development of approaches that emphasise the teaching of practical (instrumental) problem-solving skills.

Finally, an important theme taken up mainly in the last decade has been the important role of *ruminating* as a behaviour that maintains depression, and which predisposes to further episodes. It has become clear that a 'ruminative response style' – that is, responding to lowered mood by focusing your attention down onto your own thoughts and feelings – is such a risk factor (Nolen-Hoeksema and Morrow, 1991). Those who ruminate often believe that by doing so they will gain further insight and that it will help them to solve their problems, whereas in fact it has been shown to lower mood and impair problem-solving abilities (Lyubomirsky and Nolen-Hoeksema, 1995). A major approach to the reduction of risk for future episodes of depression in those at risk has been to reduce this ruminative style through the use of 'mindfulness-based CBT' (Segal *et al*, 2002).

Assessment and formulation

The following categories of information need to be sought regarding depression:

- *the presenting features*: This should include an assessment of the key biological symptoms of depression such as impaired appetite and sleep patterns. An assessment for *suicidal thoughts and intent* must always be carried out
- any *precipitating life events* or *ongoing stressors* that have played a role in causing the depression – did they come on at the same time as the depression? Is there a *family history* of depression, so that there may be a genetic predisposition, or the client may have witnessed a family member with depression and formed strong beliefs about it
- the main *cognitive markers of depression* – what are the key presenting *negative automatic thoughts (NATs)*. What do these suggest are the underlying dysfunctional assumptions and *schemas* of this patient? Is there evidence of a *negative triad of depression* and is there *depressive rumination*? How do these interrelate with the client's mood and behaviours?
- *the effects of the depression*: in particular we need to look for *reduction in pleasurable and rewarding* activities such as exercise. There may also be new *unhelpful behaviours* such as violence, gambling, or overeating
- the status of *current drug use* (including prescribed drugs) and *other health conditions*, particularly pre-existing anxiety and personality problems and medical conditions such as hypothyroidism
- the patient's *predominant coping methods*: how appropriate/successful are they? Does the patient try to worry or 'ruminate' themselves out of feeling low?

Example

Josie is a 64-year-old woman who 'lost' her husband to prostate cancer four years ago. She does not spend a significant part of her time ruminating about Ernie or his death. She has, however, found the transition to single life very difficult. Ernie, her deceased husband, had been a few years older and had organised the 'running of the house' and the couple's friends tended to be other married couples. Josie finds it difficult meeting with them now that she is 'not part of a couple'. For about 18 months Josie has felt increasingly tearful. It started when she retired from her job as a clothes-shop assistant. She wakes 'in tears and feeling shaky' at about 4 am each morning. She cries throughout the day and has lost 5 kg in weight over the last 6 months.

Generally she feels a bit better late in the evening. She can no longer be bothered with housework and is ashamed of the state of her house. She presumes that if her friends saw her house they would 'see how lazy she was' and 'would not want to know her'. She repeatedly states that her husband's death and her difficulty coping have shown just how lazy she is and how 'defective' she really has been all of her life. She no longer asks people to her house. After her retirement ex-workmates had called but she now avoids them as well. Josie avoids her sister for the same reason. She says that since she was a child, her mother (deceased for many years) had repeated a rule that 'if everyone looked after themselves then everyone would be looked after'. Josie is ashamed that Ernie had done so much and that she is now struggling. She believes that her sister would 'despair' and probably 'shout at' Josie if she knew how she was living. Josie is not aware of anyone in her family who had ever suffered with depression. Although hopeless at times, her religious beliefs prevent her from killing herself and she denies having had suicidal ideation. She has taken three antidepressant medications since becoming unwell. She has never taken illicit drugs and 'drinks only at Christmas'.

A *formulation* integrating the above information into a cognitive behavioural framework could be:

Josie has clear features of depression, including biological features such as early-morning wakening and depressed mood. She has corresponding cognitive features including a negative view of herself as lazy, the future as hopeless, and the world in the form of her negative view of her friends and family. She also engages in depressive rumination. She has emotional features of depression in the form of ongoing profound sadness and shame, and behaviourally she has reduced her activity levels, stopped cleaning the house and avoids the company of others. She appears to experience negative automatic thoughts about how she is failing by not being able to look after herself. These relate to dysfunctional assumptions that Josie has picked up from her family that to be looked after by others is a sign of weakness. Her stated schemas are that she believes herself to be lazy and defective, which are associated with strong feelings of shame. Predisposing factors include these strong dysfunctional assumptions/schemas that have been activated by her difficulties coping with practical tasks after her husband's death, and by the fact that her friendships tended to be reliant on socialising as a couple. The death of the husband may have been a precipitating factor, although Josie's mood has really deteriorated since her retirement. This deterioration may be due to the protective effect of employment in terms of reinforcing self-worth and the social contacts that she had in this role. Predominant maintaining factors include her use of depressive ruminations that lead to a deterioration in her sadness and shame. Her predominant coping mechanism has been of avoidance, resulting in reduced contact with others. Her reduced contact reminds her that in her eyes she is 'defective' and indeed not worthy of their contact. Her use of avoidance has also reduced her pleasurable and rewarding activities, another maintaining factor.

The treatment

After *socialising the client to the model*, the therapist and client need to choose the *goals of therapy*. Therefore, to some extent the approach taken will depend on these goals. Common goals are: to return to work, to assist with impaired sleep, to help the client regain contact with lost friends (lost through avoidance).

The general plan for CBT for depression is frequently as follows:

- *psycho-education* about depression. This will often include an explanation of the features of depression (including *normalising* them as understandable and relatively common). It may also include discussion around the role of medication and the importance of *medication concordance*
- generally behavioural activation approaches are tried before attempting cognitive restructuring. The initial intervention is frequently to gauge the activity levels of the client using an *activity diary*. An example is shown in Chapter 6. The client fills in how he or she filled each hour of the day over an agreed period – usually the week in between sessions. Frequently this shows that the client is spending long periods being inactive, and using unhelpful behaviours such drinking alcohol to excess. An activity diary can suggest goals for treatment and set a baseline from which to gauge change
- if the activity diary shows a reduction of activities that previously would have given a sense of reward, in particular a sense of pleasure and mastery, then *activity scheduling* is warranted. The patient may need to be coached in *reward planning* and indeed in how to self-reward in the first place. If the patient has vastly reduced activity levels, then activities may need to be re-introduced gradually in a structured and planned way – a process referred to as '*graded task assignment*'
- cognitive restructuring can then be addressed using *guided discovery* and *thought diaries* as described in Chapter 6. *Behavioural experiments* can also be used to checkout the validity of predictions and beliefs. For example, a patient's prediction that not going to bed for three hours every afternoon will worsen their mood and exhaustion levels can be tested. The patient can make subjective ratings of tiredness and mood on pre-arranged days on which they do and do not go to bed in the afternoon. Does the predicted outcome occur, and does this support or reject the hypothesis that three hours in bed daily is necessary to avoid worsening mood and exhaustion?
- *training in problem solving* will play a major part in the CBT of some patients whose poor problem-solving skills appear to have contributed to their depressed state. As part of this general approach, some people specifically benefit from training in *social skills* and *assertiveness*
- more recently developed techniques for reducing relapse in those at risk of repeated episodes of depression include '*mindfulness' training*, which helps to

keep the patient's focus in the present rather than being engaged in excessive self-focus and rumination (Segal *et al*, 2002). This is not an acute treatment for depression, but rather is used between episodes to decrease vulnerability to further episodes

- where the negative schemas are prominent, these may need addressing in their own right. This will increase the length of treatment significantly. Such *'schema-work'* is addressed in Chapter 15 of this book. It is important to note, however, that negative schemas may be prominent in many people, not just in those who may be classed as 'personality disordered'
- *relapse prevention work* in depression normally involves noting down *risk factors* and *early-warning signs* for depressive episodes. The patient and therapist then agree upon the strategies to be used should these signs re-surface. This *relapse-prevention plan* is written down and kept safe for future consultation and putting into practice as necessary. The general approach in depression is the same as that described for bipolar disorder (Chapter 8 of this book).

Josie decided that a key goal would be to learn more about depression. Her second goal was that she wanted her low mood to be alleviated, and her third was that she wanted to 'go out with friends and family' (as much as she had done before her husband's death). At the assessment the therapist had been satisfied that Josie's presentation was a consequence more of coping with the practical difficulties related to her husband's death rather than due to a problem with the grieving process. After Josie had found out more about depression – mostly via homework reading tasks, she agreed to start to look at the second goal. An activity diary was completed for three consecutive weeks. There were very few pleasurable activities written down in her diary, and there were very few times when she had contact with other people. It was clear that Josie really was avoiding social activities and that a large proportion of the day was being spend ruminating about how much of a 'mess' she had become. Josie agreed to schedule activities for the following fortnight. This included a gradual increase in social activities from a short coffee with a close friend up to a busy party three weeks later. During this graded task assignment, Josie agreed to keep a thought diary to look at some of her NATs. She gathered thoughts including: 'they think I look a mess' and: 'they want me to leave'. The latter thought, 'they want me to leave', was challenged by Josie politely asking her cousins if they needed her to leave. From their response she realised that she had misread the situation and that they did not (a behavioural experiment). She began to make use of thought diaries and began in time to challenge some of her unhelpful thoughts. She then learned more about problem solving and assertiveness techniques with the therapist, and read about financial issues, which gave her more confidence. Her mood lifted slowly, and after about 18 sessions she noticed that she had much more energy and was enjoying the company of others once again. She was discharged with a clear idea of warning signs of becoming unwell, and a plan to put into practice should her symptoms come back.

MAIN POINTS

- Beck's cognitive model of depression (Beck, *et al* 1979) describes three major concepts: the 'negative cognitive triad of depression', 'cognitive errors', and the concept of the 'schema'.
- There are many types of 'cognitive error', including 'arbitrary inference', and 'dichotomous thinking'. Williams has translated many of these into patient-friendly terms such as 'putting a negative slant on things', and 'taking a gloomy view of the future'.
- Negative schemas form mainly in childhood, and their presence has been linked with attachment problems.
- Generally, behavioural techniques addressing activity levels are used before cognitive restructuring in the treatment of depression.
- Reduced activity levels are common in depression, and are addressed using activity diaries and then activity schedules to plan activities in the week ahead.
- Activity diaries measure activities that give a sense of mastery (achievement) and pleasure.
- Challenging cognitive errors and addressing ruminating occur later in therapy using thought diaries. Mindfulness is increasingly being incorporated – particularly for the treatment of recurrent depression, alongside other relapse prevention work.

Further reading

- Beck AT, Rush AJ, Shaw B and Emery G (1979) *Cognitive Therapy of Depression.* New York: Guilford.
- Williams C (2001) *Overcoming Depression: a five areas approach.* London: Arnold.

Chapter 8

Cognitive behavioural therapy applied to bipolar disorder

The models • Assessment and formulation • The treatment

The models

Beck, 1967 described the symptoms of mania in similar but opposite terms to those of depression. Therefore, he spoke of the *'negative cognitive triad' of depression* and the *'positive cognitive triad' of mania*. Instead of an overly negative view of the self, world and future, he said that manic patients hold an overly positive view of these three areas. They may view themselves as excessively capable, the world in glowing rosy terms and the future as opportune with few potential problems or obstacles. In the same way that Beck surmised that depressed patients have *depressed cognitive distortions* such as selectively abstracting the negative aspects of a situation, he saw manic patients exhibiting similar but opposite *manic cognitive distortions*. For example, the positive aspects of a situation may be selectively concentrated upon, and the risks ignored.

Patients' behaviours have been found to influence the likelihood of experiencing an affective episode (Lam and Wong 1997). Indeed, bipolar disorder (BD) is now viewed as an example of a *'diathesis-stress disorder'* (Goodwin and Jamison, 1990; Lam *et al*, 1999). This means that there may be an underlying, biological vulnerability to the disorder, but an episode may not be precipitated unless other environmental factors are present such as stress, life events or illicit substance misuse. This biological vulnerability may be due to *'circadian rhythm instability'* (Healy and Williams, 1989). Circadian rhythms are hormone-driven functions that vary in a predictable manner through the day. The sleep–wake cycle is a good example. BD clients may respond to 'stresses' to their circadian rhythms by becoming unwell. Irregular food intake and sleep disturbance are examples of such 'stresses'. The influence of stress on the BD client can be reduced by medications such as *'mood stabilisers'*.

Another key element in the cognitive behavioural understanding of bipolar disorder is the *'prodrome'*. This refers to warning features such as talking less or staying late at work that indicate that a patient is progressively moving towards an affective episode. It is also important to note that although the features of a prodrome differ significantly between individuals, a given patient is likely to exhibit the same or similar prodromal features during each episode of illness. This has been termed their *'relapse signature'* (Smith and Tarrier, 1992). Therefore, prodromes warn that a patient is moving towards an episode of illness, and we know that what happens to the patient during this crucial time influences whether they experience an episode or not. A key role of CBT is to influence outcomes by influencing the actions of the patient during their prodromes (Basco and Rush, 1996; Lam *et al*, 1999; Scott, 2001).

The model of Lam *et al* (1999) proposes that those with a biological vulnerability to BD will move into prodromal stages, but whether they progress into a formal episode of illness will be influenced by their *coping styles*. Unhelpful coping styles such as reducing activities in depression or increasing them during hypomania can precipitate an episode, and cause the client's mood state to deteriorate once in an episode. Lam *et al* (1999) state that the stigma and relationship problems that are common consequences of the client's behaviours when unwell add to other stresses such as life events and periods of sleep disturbance. All of these factors then interact with their biological vulnerability.

Scott *et al* (2000) have also found that bipolar populations have *poor problem-solving skills* as well as fragile and unstable levels of self-esteem. Both of these areas may be potential targets for change.

Assessment and formulation

The following are pointers towards some of the information that needs to be gathered for bipolar disorder:

- an assessment of *current symptoms* of an affective disorder. Don't forget mixed affective states where, for example, you may have racing thoughts and elated mood but reduced activity levels. As always check for *modifiers* of the symptoms – that is, what makes the symptoms worse and what makes them better?
- as thoroughly as possible assess for episodes of high and low mood through the patient's life thus far. Are there *patterns* where symptom clusters come on together?
- is there evidence of *prodromal features* of both the high and the low episodes? Do these remain constant for each episode – that is, is there a *relapse signature*? How do the episodes progress? What circumstances appear to *precipitate* the episodes, e.g. excess stress and stimulation?
- what has the client used to try and *cope* with their symptoms and how successful have they been? For example, have they responded to hypomania by allowing themselves to increase their activity levels?
- what have been the *consequences* of these previous episodes? What has been the *effect of the episodes* on the patient's life and view of themselves? In particular, look at evidence of *loss*, perhaps in terms of employment or relationships
- what is the client's attitude towards and compliance with *prescribed medication*?
- assess for *co-morbid mental health problems* – in particular substance misuse and personality problems.

Example

Ian is a 29-year-old landscape gardener. Currently, he has increased activity levels, slight pressure of speech and reduced sleep requirement (4 hours).

There are no psychotic phenomena. He has 'renewed energy for life and self-confidence', and after having been single for some years is dating two women. He says he 'looks great'. He has also started to feel very confident in his job, putting himself forward for a promotion. Ian has only had two obvious previous episodes of illness (both hypomanic). These resulted in him having to 'give up good jobs'. Prior to both previous episodes of hypomania, Ian had broken up with 'serious girlfriends'. Less than one month after each break-up he began to 'find work easier'. He needed less sleep and finally began to engage in risky behaviours such as driving his car at speed. When well he complies with medication. Currently Ian wants to come off lithium. When high, Ian just 'goes with the flow'. He takes his music system up to his room and gets 'high on "heavy metal" music'. He also stops his lithium. Being high has had a marked impact on Ian's life, although on recovering from previous episodes Ian generally copes well with life without apparent stigma for his illness or low self-esteem. He does not drink or use drugs.

A *formulation* could include the following:

Ian has bipolar disorder. He is currently hypomanic and he exhibits features of Beck's positive cognitive triad. In particular, he holds an overly positive 'grandiose' view of himself and the future. His predominant coping mechanism when high is to allow himself to 'go with the flow' and to listen to loud music. He also ceases to comply with the suggested medication regime. There is no evidence that he has enough insight to try and consciously reduce his activity levels when high. These strategies probably cause his mood to become further elevated. There is therefore a vicious circle of increasing elation driven by unhelpful behaviours. Ian appears to have a clear prodromal 'relapse signature', which includes the feature of finding his work progressively easier than normally is the case. His subsequent symptoms also form a characteristic progression from a reduced need for sleep, culminating in engaging in risky behaviours.

The treatment

The diathesis-stress model of bipolar disorder (as described) has resulted in CBT approaches tending to integrate a variety of psychosocial and medication-based treatments. This requires collaboration between a variety of health workers as well as family members. The message given to the client is that *CBT is an adjunct to medication rather than an alternative* (Scott, 2001).

- *Psycho-education*: the diathesis-stress model and the importance of keeping regular routines to minimise circadian rhythm disruption are normally discussed.
- *Identify and monitor mood symptoms*: helping the client to identify and rate the severity of their symptoms is one of the most important elements of treatment.

The 'card-sorting technique' (Perry *et al*, 1999) can be used. Here the general features of mood disorders (e.g. sleeping less, tearfulness) are listed one symptom per card. The client looks through the cards and separates out those that apply to them when they are high and when they are low. Once the general features have been identified, the client begins to decide upon those features that occur at different levels of illness severity. So called *'anchor points'* (Scott, 2001) can be used to link illness features with the severity of illness by constructing a scale from −10 through zero and up to +10. The minus figures correspond with depression, so that −10 is most depressed, and the positive figures correspond to the client's hypomania/mania so that +10 corresponds to the most elated point that the client has ever experienced. In Table 8.1, only the anchor points of 0 to +10 have been used as the client had not previously been depressed. Once the anchor points have been identified, the client can *practise plotting their daily mood score* that corresponds to each anchor point. For example, they may allocate and plot a score of −4 one day, as −4 corresponds to feeling low in motivation and tearful. The next day they may allocate themselves a score of −2 as they have distracted themselves, feel slightly more motivated and are not tearful. Plotting these daily mood scores over time builds up a *'mood chart'* (Scott, 2001). Mood charts illustrate those factors that have an impact on the client's mood. To minimise mood changes in the future, the client can then attend to these factors.

- *Identify risk factors using a 'life chart'*: in a similar way that mood charts illustrate the influences on the client's mood over days to weeks, a life chart does the same but looks back over the life span of the client. Previous episodes are plotted with time along the *x* axis and severity of illness along the *y* axis. The therapist and

Table 8.1 Ian's 'anchor points' (for more information on 'anchor points', *see* Scott, 2001)

Anchor Point	My features at that anchor point
+10	'Joy riding' through the night. Sexually suggestive comments to women ++
+9	Speak very fast. Very flirtatious
+8	Give up going into work. Going to nightclubs nightly
+7	Going to nightclubs in the week, have confidence to chat up women, may sleep less than 3–4 hours
+6	Nightclubs at weekend, offering lifts to workmates, making lots of plans for 'projects'
+5	Sleep less than 5 hours nightly; begin to think more about changing jobs or getting new 'project'
+4	Talk to people at work about getting a 'raise'
+3	Sleep less than 6.5 hours a night
+2	Work begins to be 'easy'
+1	Feel happy in the mornings
0	Life going on as normal

client can decide to add any influence to the chart, although life events and medication changes are most frequently added to show the impact of these on becoming unwell.

- *Using prodromes*: clients are encouraged to identify (perhaps through consultation with friends and family) those early warning signs of both going high and becoming depressed (Lam *et al*, 1999). It is important that the therapist and client write down for easy consultation appropriate coping strategies to use should the early warning signs become apparent. For example, if the client notices that they are retreating into themselves (an early-warning sign of depression), then an appropriate coping strategy might be to plan an activity schedule.
- *Specific strategies to be used during an episode of depression*: these are the same as those outlined in Chapter 7 of this book, on depression.
- *Specific strategies to be used during an episode of hypomania*: generally, these tactics either attempt to reduce the likelihood of negative consequences from being elated, or *reduce stimulation levels*, thus preventing deterioration in the elated mood state. '*Delay tactics*' such as the '48 hour rule' have been used to prevent the client acting impulsively with negative consequences. The client agrees a rule whereby any major decision or action is delayed by 48 hours to allow them to consider the consequences before they act. Similarly, they may agree to a 'two-person rule'. This requires the client to speak with two trusted confidantes about the plans or actions before they act. Although the '48 hour rule' was originally described by Aaron T. Beck, a variety of 'delay tactics' are described by Scott (2001).
- *Encourage medication concordance*: the life chart frequently shows that previous episodes have been associated with stopping mood stabilisers. Listing the advantages and disadvantages of taking the medication versus not taking the medication can also make the situation clearer.
- *Dealing with underlying problems*: there may be serious issues that increase the vulnerability of the client to further illness episodes, including substance misuse problems, social isolation or stigma.

The first treatment sessions introduced Ian to the diathesis-stress model, emphasising the fact that behaviours had an impact on the progression of the illness. Ian constructed anchor points for his hypomania (*see* Table 8.1), and practised rating his mood. Ian also agreed to experiment with not listening to loud music. On the days that he did not give into the urge to 'plug himself in', he found that his subsequent mood normalised from +7 to +5. At session 6, Ian's mood had fallen to a level of +1 or +2. Now he was better able to consider the factors that had contributed to him becoming unwell in the past. Ian and the therapist did this by spending two sessions constructing a 'life chart'. This reinforced the finding that stopping lithium in the past had predicted subsequent relapse. He therefore decided to continue his medication. Specific strategies for hypomania were further addressed. The '48 hour rule' and the 'two-person rule' were discussed. Ian thought that both were good ideas and wrote out these rules on 'flashcards', which he put into a separate pocket in his wallet. His mood was noted to be at the 'zero' or 'normal' point after 14 sessions. His mother attended the next session and the three constructed a list of warning signs of becoming high, together with a detailed plan should they occur. Ian and his mother did not agree on the significance of all of the signs, but agreed upon a core list of eight early-warning signs, separating them into 'early', 'middle' and 'late' ones. The coping plan differed for each of the three categories. For example, if he showed 'late early-warning signs', such as 'repeatedly talking fast about work' then there was a written agreement that an urgent appointment would be sought with Ian's CPN.

MAIN POINTS

- Beck described the 'positive cognitive triad of mania' referring to thoughts regarding an overly positive view of the self, world and the future. There are similar but opposite forms of cognitive distortions or errors to those seen in depression, such as minimising risk.
- Bipolar disorder (BD) is an example of a 'diathesis-stress disorder', that is a disorder which is influenced by both underlying biological vulnerability and precipitating environmental factors for its expression.
- CBT for BD should be provided in addition to rather than as an alternative to medication.
- Circadian rhythm instability may be a key factor in the causation of BD. It is also key in the treatment, by attempting to minimise disruptions to daily life.
- The ability to identify and change the risk factors for experiencing episodes of depression and mania is a key part of treatment. This involves practising identifying and then acting upon the 'prodromes' of illness episodes. These can be identified by exploring past episodes in the patient's life using a 'life chart'.

Further reading

- Lam DH, Jones SH, Hayward P and Bright JA (1999) *Cognitive Therapy for Bipolar Disorder: a therapist's guide to concepts, methods and practice.* Chichester: Wiley.
- Scott J (2001) *Overcoming Mood Swings.* New York: New York University Press.

Chapter 9

Cognitive behavioural therapy applied to phobias and panic

The models • Assessment and formulation • The treatment

The models

The same thinking errors that occur in depression also occur in anxiety disorders. However, the predominant content of the cognitions seen in anxiety disorders relates to *threat* rather than to *loss* (Beck and Clark, 1988). Specifically, cognitive behavioural theories of anxiety state that sufferers tend to *overestimate the threat* of given situations and they tend to *underestimate their own ability to cope* with those situations (Beck and Clark, 1988). The feared 'situation' may be limited to a discrete 'threat' such as for simple phobias, or may be much more generalised such as with panic disorder (PD) and generalised anxiety disorder (GAD).

In simple phobias (such as spider phobias) the client's perception of threat may have its origin in earlier experiences – perhaps being stung by an insect in childhood. There may also be an 'inbuilt' biological propensity to be fearful of spiders. In addition, the phobic may also have learned that spiders are dangerous through observing the phobias of others, adding to the *association* made between the client and the *feared stimulus* (in this case the spider). Their repeated *avoidance* of the feared stimulus maintains the phobia by *operant conditioning*. That is, over time they learn that avoidance reduces their unpleasant anxiety symptoms so that they are more likely to avoid more and more in the future. By avoiding the feared stimulus they also fail to learn that it is not as dangerous as they presume.

The cognitive model of *panic disorder* proposed by Clark (1986a) outlines three major processes that then maintain the disorder once it has started. One process is the *'catastrophic misinterpretation of bodily sensations'*. This means that panic sufferers tend to use the thinking error of 'catastrophisation' in relation to bodily sensations. In particular, normal and harmless symptoms of anxiety, such as an awareness of the heart beating fast, are interpreted as evidence of impending disaster. Table 9.1 shows how some normal anxiety symptoms are misinterpreted in panic. Commonly in panic the thoughts happen in pictures in the sufferer's mind (*imagery*). They not only believe that they are going to collapse or have a heart attack, or even die, but they can see it happening in their 'mind's eye'. Clark proposed that the effect of these catastrophic thoughts and images is that the individual becomes even more anxious. The more anxious they become, the more they have the fast heart, the dizziness, the tingling fingers – which are further interpreted as evidence

Table 9.1 Anxiety features and typical catastrophic misinterpretations in panic

Anxiety feature	Typical misinterpretation of that feature in panic
Awareness of heart beating fast	'I'm having a heart attack'
Feeling dizzy/light-headed	'I'll faint and collapse'
Dissociation	'I'm losing control/going mad'
Tingling in fingers	'I'm going to die'

of impending disaster. That is, the individual gets into a vicious circle of anxiety features and catastrophisation. Sometimes other sensations such as palpitations associated with caffeine intake rather than anxiety *per se* are the initial 'seeds' that are misinterpreted. These then cause anxiety features in exactly the same way, starting the vicious circle and the panic attack.

Another process proposed by Clark is *'hyper-vigilance'*. This refers to the fact that panic sufferers tend to carefully watch out or *scan* for these feared anxiety features. They are so attentive that they frequently pick up on sensations that they would otherwise fail to even notice. Therefore, not only do they react more strongly and catastrophically to these features, but they also pick up on more of them in the first place.

The third process that appears to maintain panic disorder is the use of *'safety behaviours'* and *'avoidance'*. With reference to panic these can be categorised into three main areas (Salkovskis, 1996):

1. avoiding the feared situation in the first place, e.g. never travelling on public transport
2. running away or escaping from a situation during an episode of panic
3. using other, often quite subtle, safety behaviours during the panic attack to prevent the feared catastrophe, e.g. sitting down and clinging onto the chair to avoid fainting.

All three forms of avoidance and safety behaviour described above prevent the client from finding out that the threat is not so great after all (Salkovskis, 1996). So, the client who always clings to the supermarket shopping trolley, for fear that unless they do they will faint, never has this presumption challenged. If they never test this presumption out it will become stronger over time with repeated episodes of panic. They can always tell themselves 'thankfully I didn't faint because I was able to hold on to the trolley'.

Assessment and formulation

The following information will normally be sought regarding *phobias*:

- what is the client actually afraid of? The precise characteristics of the *'feared object'* and the *'feared consequences'* of contact with the feared object need to be described in as much detail as possible. For example, if the fear is of spiders, what is it about spiders that is frightening? Is it all spiders or just large ones, or perhaps small ones that jump? What do they imagine happening? Do they fear being stung? What do they fear would happen even if they were stung?

- are there times or circumstances when the situation/feared object is *more or less frightening*?
- when did the phobia *start*, and what was happening in the client's life when it started? How has the phobia *developed* over time?
- how does the client try and cope with the phobia – specifically do they use *safety behaviours and avoidance*?

Similarly, for *panic*:

- *what happens* during a panic attack? Remember to use the 'five-areas model' (Williams, 2001). What happens afterwards? Are there patterns in terms of the features that come on first?
- what is the *client afraid will happen* during a panic attack – the *feared consequences*? For example, what do they think is the significance of the palpitations? What is their evidence that the feared consequence(s) will happen?
- we need to know the events that lead up to the panic attacks, and the situations and times in which the attacks occur – *the precipitants*
- is there something that the client particularly *fears* independent of the panicking itself? In particular, are there associated features of agoraphobia – so that the client is afraid of open spaces, crowded situations and the scrutiny of others?
- what has the client used to try and cope with the panic; in particular do they use *avoidance and safety behaviours*?
- finally, what is the status of current *drug use* (including prescribed drugs such as benzodiazepines) and other *mental health conditions*, particularly depression?

Example

Anne is a 43-year-old woman who said that she had always felt very uneasy being among large groups of people. She feared that she would be shown to be 'different or silly in some way' and potentially humiliated. She remembers being stared at when she froze and 'made a fool' of herself during a school drama production. Her first formal panic attack, however, was only two years ago. She remembers feeling sweaty, dizzy and ill when buying a newspaper in a newsagent's shop. She also remembers thinking that she was going to collapse in the shop. Her panic attacks became more and more frequent, and are currently preventing her from leaving her home (except during the night, when she believes it will be very quiet). A typical attack comprises an awareness of her heart racing, sweating, dizziness and difficulty 'catching her breath'. She does have the attacks at home alone now even though they initially occurred only in crowded places. They now occur at any time of day. During an attack she stays as still as possible, hoping that this will make her heart slow down and also lessen her chances of fainting. She listens for her heart rate, fearing that it will get ever faster, ultimately 'seizing up' and stopping, resulting in her death. She is not depressed and does not take any medication or illicit drugs.

A *formulation* may include:

> Anne has schemas relating to others as 'threatening' and to herself as 'vulnerable' that act as a predisposing factor to the development of her symptoms of anxiety and panic. She has typical symptoms of agoraphobia and panic. She has a variety of physical features of panic, and misinterprets her fast heartbeat as evidence of further threat in the form of a heart attack followed by death. She scans her body for other evidence of an ensuing heart attack, which feeds back to further increase her symptoms of anxiety. These are further misinterpreted as evidence of threat, resulting in a vicious circle. Her predominant mode of coping has been to avoid most social situations, leading to a significantly impaired quality of life and isolation. She also uses safety behaviours in the form of trying to remain motionless, believing that this prevents the feared consequence of having a heart attack. She has never stopped herself from carrying out this behaviour and therefore has never had reason to doubt that this truly prevents a heart attack. There is no evidence of an underlying pharmacological cause of the panic or of concurrent illness including depression.

The treatment

The underlying principle in the behavioural treatment of phobias is *'graded exposure in vivo'*. Clients are gradually exposed to the feared stimulus. There is a concurrent reduction in anxiety symptoms that occurs when the body remains in a threatening situation for a significant amount of time without the occurrence of the feared consequence – that is they become *'habituated'* to the threat. They also learn that the threat from it is not as great as they had previously believed. The exposure can take the form of the client imagining the feared stimulus (*imaginal exposure*) or literally facing up to whatever it is that is feared (*exposure in vivo*). For example, spider phobics can begin their exposure programmes by imagining spiders, and this will often be enough to cause significant emotional and physical features of fear. Later they may be able to look at pictures of spiders and once they feel comfortable with these they may be able to cope with being in the presence of a real spider in the room, then within arm's length and sometimes even to touch or hold the spider. It is important that the exposure is gradually increased and that the levels of anxiety are significantly reduced (habituation) before progressing to the next level. The levels are agreed upon before the beginning of the programme of exposure, and presented as an *'exposure hierarchy'*. An exposure hierarchy for a spider phobic has just been described above – that is the progression from imaginal exposure to holding or touching a real spider. The general principle is the same for all exposure work with phobias – another exposure hierarchy is shown in Table 9.2, this time for a teacher with a phobia of public speaking. In reality the list may be more comprehensive so that there are more levels (or goals) to gradually work towards. In *social phobia*, this exposure may be supplemented with 'video feedback'. Videotaping 'social performances' and then watching the tape alongside the therapist allows the client to measure his or her true performance and to challenge

Table 9.2 Exposure hierarchy for a client (teacher) with a phobia of pubic speaking

Degree client fears the given situation (%)	Feared situation
100	Speaking in conference at Brighton
95	Giving feedback to the board at work in front of management
85	Playing my part on the first night of the pantomime
80	Talking in front of 30 parents at parents' evening
75	Giving a talk to the 20 school staff
65	Giving a talk to the 10 first year staff
55	Talking about the staff changes in the staff room to a small group
50	Talking in the assembly to the kids and one or two staff

pre-conceptions such as the extent of blushing. The use of graded exposure in vivo would be the general approach for clients who have *agoraphobia*. If they also experience panic attacks then techniques in addition to the graded exposure are used to treat the panic.

- The initial intervention is almost always to use a *'panic diary'*. This allows the collection of more detailed information about the circumstances of the panic and the effect of the treatment interventions on the frequency and intensity of the panic symptoms (Clark, 1989). Although the diaries vary, most include a note of the date and time of the panic attack, how long it lasted and the situation where it occurred. The symptoms of the attack are noted including the associated thoughts as well as some rating (normally 0–100) of how severe the attack was.

- Usually the panic diary will elucidate the *catastrophic beliefs* that help to fuel the panic attacks – that the client will collapse, have a heart attack, die, etc. These beliefs need to be challenged, and this is often achieved using *'panic induction techniques'* (Salkovskis *et al*, 1986). In essence, these techniques recreate as closely as possible some of the sensations of panic, but in a safe environment. The client learns that the sensations are not as dangerous as presumed. The most common induction technique used is *voluntary hyperventilation*. Here the client is asked to quickly over-breathe through their nose and mouth for two minutes. The effects are similar to panic in most people. The following discussion allows the client and therapist to challenge whether the light-headed feelings, the pins and needles in the fingers, and the other features present in both the induction techniques and the panic are evidence of collapse, fainting, etc. It can be discussed with the patient that the symptoms are probably due to *hypocapnia* – that is a lowered level of carbon dioxide in the blood. This is the result of blowing off too much carbon dioxide in the breath in hyperventilation. Usually the patient does not feel that they were hyperventilating. It is important to point out that at rest we naturally breathe in and out only very small volumes of air. Therefore, despite the subjective feeling that they can not get enough air into their lungs they are actually more than likely to be taking in far more air than would normally be the case. Note that voluntary hyperventilation should not be carried out if there are medical concerns such as asthma, chronic obstructive pulmonary disease (COPD), epilepsy or pregnancy, and if the CBT is being carried out by a non-medical practitioner then a medical assessment is recommended before attempting voluntary hyperventilation.

- The discussion around panic induction can be supplemented with the use of *education materials*, which provide a written record to remind the client in the future. The education material might include issues such as the fact that panic causes an increased blood pressure that reduces rather increases the chances of fainting (despite the sensations that resemble those of fainting).

- If it is agreed that hyperventilation results in the sensations of panic for the client, then they can be taught the method of '*controlled respiration*'. This involves slow (not more than 12 breaths per minute) and shallow breathing, using the abdomen rather than using the chest wall (Clark, 1986b; Salkovskis *et al*, 1986). It is important to note that in common with relaxation, controlled respiration can be misused as a 'safety behaviour'. For this reason its use is again debated within CBT.

- As panic patients believe that they are protected by their *avoidance and safety behaviours*, these need to be stopped (Salkovskis, 1996). The avoidance can be addressed using *graded exposure in vivo* if necessary. The client also progressively drops the safety behaviours, as a behavioural experiment. Subsequent discussion usually shows that they had not indeed been preventing 'the worst' from happening.

After two weeks of completing a 'panic diary' it became clear that Anne's panic attacks always occurred after she had been thinking about having a heart attack. The key belief was that her breathing and her heart rate would rise out of control, resulting in a heart attack. She carried out an experiment at home where she counted her heart rate during a panic attack at 114 beats per minute. When she did the same when carrying out a fast walk her heart rate was almost the same, despite feeling relatively relaxed – obviously the heart happily coped with these high rates! This helped to challenge her belief that panicking would cause a heart attack. Then the client consented to try voluntary hyperventilation. This proved to be distressing for Anne who stated that the sensations were identical to those she experienced in her panic. She also held onto her chest and stayed perfectly still in the session, therefore playing out her safety behaviours in front of the therapist. Afterwards, the therapist explained why there was such a similarity in sensations between the induction and her panic attacks and also began to look at what causes heart attacks and, equally, what does not. Anne experimented with keeping moving while panicking (stopping her safety behaviour of staying still), and noted that this did not cause problems. Finally, Anne's agoraphobia was addressed, with the creation of an exposure hierarchy. Gradually, she went out of the house, firstly in the early evening to local shops and then to a nearby supermarket in the afternoon. With practice she was able to function in the supermarket despite mild self-consciousness.

MAIN POINTS

- Patients with anxiety disorders overestimate threat and underestimate their ability to cope with it.
- Phobic patients fail to learn that the feared stimulus is not as dangerous as they presume. Their repeated avoidance of the feared stimulus maintains the phobia by operant conditioning.
- Clark's model of panic disorder (Clark, 1986a) states that three major processes maintain it: the catastrophic misinterpretation of bodily sensations, hypervigilance, and the use of safety behaviours and avoidance.
- Safety behaviours can be subtle and difficult to identify, but stopping them is essential to allow full exposure and habituation to the feared stimulus.
- Exposure is a key treatment element in anxiety disorders. In phobias, an exposure hierarchy is constructed and the patient is exposed in a graded way to situations that provoke progressively more anxiety. Habituation to the feared stimulus is the aim of exposure.
- Panic-induction techniques such as voluntary hyperventilation help to educate that the physical symptoms of panic are understandable, predictable and preventable.
- Voluntary hyperventilation should be carried out with care and not used with patients who are pregnant or have respiratory or cardiac problems. Non-medical practitioners should seek medical advice before attempting voluntary hyperventilation.

Further reading

- Clark DM (1989) Anxiety states: panic and generalised anxiety. In: Hawton K, Salkovskis PM, Kirk J and Clark DM (eds) *Cognitive Behaviour Therapy*. Oxford: Oxford University Press, pp. 52–96.
- Salkovskis PM (1991) The importance of behaviour in the maintenance of anxiety and panic: a cognitive account. *Behavioural Psychotherapy* **19**: 6–19.

Chapter 10

Cognitive behavioural therapy applied to generalised anxiety disorder

---

The models • Assessment and formulation • The treatment

The models

As previously stated anxiety sufferers tend to *overestimate the threat* of given situations and *underestimate their own ability to cope* with those situations (Beck and Clark, 1988). In generalised anxiety disorder (GAD) this hypervigilance to threat occurs throughout the day rather than only at times when the sufferer is faced with a specific feared object, as is the case for phobias. This view of the world as threatening and of themselves as vulnerable (schemas or core beliefs) may be related to insecure attachment patterns in childhood (Riskind *et al*, 2004). The way that panic or phobic patients cope with the perception of threat is to avoid the specific feared object – be that spiders, crowded places, etc. GAD sufferers commonly avoid a much wider range of situations that they view as threatening.

A crucial element of GAD is *worry*. Sufferers often use worry to avoid or prepare themselves to cope with future threat (Beck *et al*, 1985). However, GAD sufferers typically hold conflicting views about worry. These are brought together in *Wells' model of GAD* (Wells, 1997). They may view worrying as essential to prepare themselves for threat. As a group they engage in worrying to a much greater degree than the general population, worrying mainly about *future events that could go wrong*. These worries about 'external' issues are termed *'type 1 worry'* by Wells. GAD sufferers also commonly worry about the worrying activity in itself (worry about worry). Commonly they believe that their worry could go out of control and that this could end up with them 'totally losing control' or 'going mad'. This worry about worry has been termed *'type 2 worry'* or *'meta-worry'*. As well as thoughts, some GAD sufferers experience catastrophic *imagery*, which also results in intense feelings of fear.

People with GAD also commonly believe that viewing events in the most negative way possible is a benefit – 'It can't get any worse than this, so if I'm prepared for that then I'll be prepared for anything' (Borkovec, 1994). Their thoughts are biased towards the most negative and catastrophic outcomes. Furthermore, many worriers 'play out' in their mind as many possible threat scenarios as possible, despite there being little evidence that any will actually occur. This has been termed *'what-iffing'* behaviour (Kendall and Ingram, 1987). Unfortunately, when engaged in these worries, to some extent it is as if those negative events are truly happening. Worrying therefore results in *physiological features of anxiety* (tenseness, chronic low-grade hyperventilation, etc). It can also result in feelings of *hopelessness* and *depression* as well as tiredness and exhaustion from the worry and resulting impaired sleep.

Assessment and formulation

The following information will normally be sought regarding GAD:

- what are the *presenting features of anxiety*? As always it will be useful to map out a *five-areas assessment*
- what factors *modulate* the anxiety – that is what makes it better and what makes it worse?
- what are the contents of the patient's worries (*type 1 worries*)?
- what are the client's beliefs about worrying – do they see worrying as necessary, as a threat or as both (*type 2 worries*)?
- what is *actually happening in the client's life* in relation to these worries – i.e. to what degree are the worries understandable in the context of the client's life, is there a clear *precipitating factor*? Are there *previous episodes* of similar anxiety and what precipitated these episodes?
- is the anxiety long-standing, or are there *other factors* that explain the anxiety at this time – e.g. illicit drugs, depressive disorder, or another anxiety disorder such as panic disorder.

Example

Jonathan described himself as always having been 'nervy'. He had been bullied in school and thought it was best never to get too close to others or they would 'take advantage of you'. He felt anxious for most of the day, most days. His major symptoms of anxiety were light-headedness, palpitations, concentration problems and constantly feeling tired. He described worrying about the future – in particular that he might fail in his job as a computer technician. He worried that he might get something wrong and that the computer system would be damaged by his actions, ending up with significant financial loss for the company. He described a 'picture in his mind' of his boss telling him about this damage, that he was looking at the ground with a look of shame on his face. He also believed that at times when he became 'upset' he found it difficult to concentrate and would stop sleeping. It was at these times that he believed he might 'lose it'. He defined 'losing it' as becoming extremely anxious and feeling like he was on the verge of a nervous breakdown. He had never actually had a 'nervous breakdown'. He believed this was because he had protected himself from a breakdown by 'eventually working things out in my head'. When anxious he scans his body for evidence of moving towards 'meltdown'. The evidence that he would be looking for would be: 'pins and needles', not being able to think straight, light-headedness, saying silly things and sweating. When these start he worries that it's going to get worse and worse till he 'loses it' (has a nervous breakdown). He does not drink alcohol at all or take any drugs including caffeine believing that they would push him to have a nervous breakdown.

A *formulation* integrating the above information could be:

> Jonathan has core beliefs relating to others as 'threatening' and to himself as 'vulnerable'. These act as predisposing factors for the development of GAD. He has prominent imagery with a catastrophic content. Similarly, his thoughts are dominated by the theme that he may be threatened in the future (type 1 worry) and he exhibits the thinking styles (Williams, 2001) of catastrophising, bearing all responsibility and overgeneralising. He engages in extensive worrying, believing that this will help him to prepare him for the future. He also, however, believes that this worrying could cause him to 'lose control' and 'have a nervous breakdown' – examples of type 2 worry. He has long-standing physiological features of anxiety. These are exacerbated by his worry about the future (particularly when he perceives this as getting 'out of control'). When anxious he is hypervigilant for signs that he is losing control, and misinterprets a wide variety of physiological signs of anxiety such as light-headedness as evidence of this. He therefore finds himself trapped in a vicious circle of rising symptoms of anxiety that cause more worry, that causes more anxiety. His total avoidance of all substances including alcohol and caffeine could be conceptualised as 'safety behaviours'. There is no evidence of concurrent illness, including depression.

The treatment

Addressing the behaviour of worrying – in particular type 2 worries – has become an increasingly important element of the cognitive behavioural approach to GAD (Wells, 1997). The treatment primarily addresses the behavioural (avoidance), cognitive (worry), physiological (physical anxiety symptoms) and the imagery elements of GAD:

- in the same way that panic diaries are used to gather further details and monitor panic episodes, '*worry logs*' (Leahy and Holland, 2000) are also used to learn about the content of the client's worries and to identify the cues that precipitate their worrying. Most worry logs contain the content of the worries, the situation in which they occurred, a rating of the degree to which they were believed at the time, and the effects of the worries (e.g. increasing physical anxiety symptoms). There should also be an identification of the actual outcome – i.e. the degree to which the worries 'came true'
- some clinicians also ask the client in-session to '*worry out loud*', that is to speak along to their own stream of worrying thoughts as they go through their mind. The *biased nature of the worries* often becomes apparent at this early stage
- the *value of worrying* needs to be investigated – this will challenge the client's positive beliefs that worrying prepares them and is therefore protective. The client can list both the *advantages and the disadvantages of worrying*. The worry logs may show a wide variety of information that can be used to challenge the client's positive beliefs about worrying. A further challenge to the usefulness of worry is

to artificially *ask the client to not worry* for a period, perhaps a few days, and monitor to see whether the client was any less prepared/came to any harm

- the beliefs about the uncontrollability and the resulting dangerous effects of worrying (*type 2 worry*) can also be challenged by setting a number of other behavioural experiments. The client can be instructed to try and deliberately lose control of worry such as by asking them to repeatedly think '*what if* the worst thing happened and then the worst thing after that and so on (Wells, 1997). They find that not only do they not lose control, but also that it is not possible to prepare for all negative eventualities. *Deferring the worry* to agreed set *worry periods* can also challenge the belief about the uncontrollability of worry. For example, the therapist and client may agree a set worry period of 7–7.30 in the evening. Some clients are surprised that they are able to defer their worry (at least to a significant degree) and decide to continue worry periods if they perceive that dropping worrying completely would be too challenging

- the futility of worry can also be shown by *looking at the true probability* of some of their type 1 worries actually happening. Most overestimate the chances of events happening. If the probability of a feared event happening relies on the interaction of a number of other unlikely events, then the probability of the feared event actually occurring is a multiplication of the other small likelihoods. So if the chances of meeting the boss in the train station relies on the one in ten chance that he comes by train that day, the one in five chance that he comes on a certain train and perhaps a one in two chance that he sees the client, then the overall probability is a multiplication of these probabilities – that is only a one in a hundred chance!

- the physiological, autonomic features of anxiety can also be addressed using *relaxation training*. Likewise the use of behavioural activation and exercise can help to both relax and reduce the time available for worrying (Leahy and Holland, 2000)

- *imagery training* allows clients to imagine positive or neutral outcomes to stressful scenes as they emerge in their mind. Imagery also forms a part of relaxation training in the holding in mind of a favorite relaxing scene – perhaps a beautiful beach, that can help to induce feelings of relaxation.

Jonathan's 'worry log' showed that he had a wide variety of type 1 worries relating to threat at work. They were often related to obscure, very unlikely outcomes. Identifying all of the constituent circumstances that would need to occur, and multiplying their corresponding probabilities explored the probability of a power cut at work. Losing power would require a severe storm, a national loss of power and a failure of the company's own two generators. The overall probability of loss of power was estimated at a one in 180000 chance each weekend! None of the feared outcomes in his worry log came true, which further persuaded him that his worrying was doing him 'no favours'. His type 2 worry was addressed by getting him to 'postpone' worrying. He was able to do it during 20 minute periods in the early evening (but not at other times in the day). This allowed him to see that he could control his worrying to some extent. He practised a variety of relaxation training techniques including abdominal breathing, and used an image of a relaxing scene from his childhood on a beach on the west coast of Scotland. He accepted that he might always be prone to anxiety, but left therapy much more confident that he could intercept and prevent escalation of anxiety symptoms in the future.

MAIN POINTS

- People with GAD overestimate levels of threat in a wide variety of situations, which may be linked with insecure attachment patterns in childhood.
- Worry is a key part of GAD. Wells describes 'type 1' worry (about external threatening events), and 'type 2' worry (about one's own worrying thoughts). Imagery can also form a key part of the 'worrying'.
- Thinking styles such as 'considering the worst-case scenarios' and 'what-iffing' contribute to maintain some people's GAD.
- These styles of thinking probably also contribute to the high rates of depression seen in those with GAD.
- Identifying the content of worry and then challenging this using 'worry logs' forms a major part of therapy.
- Education about true risk and probabilities and experimentation with 'worry-free' periods help to challenge beliefs that worry is necessary and protective, and also that it cannot be controlled.
- Other non-specific stress-reduction techniques such as exercise, relaxation training, and practising imagining relaxing scenes can also be helpful.

Further reading

- Riskind JH, Williams NL, Altman MD *et al.* (2004) Parental bonding, attachment, and development of the looming maladaptive style. *Journal of Cognitive Psychotherapy: An International Quarterly* 18: 43–52.
- Wells A (1997) *Cognitive Therapy of Anxiety Disorders: a practice manual and conceptual guide*. Chichester: Wiley.

Chapter 11

Cognitive behavioural therapy applied to obsessive-compulsive disorder

The models • Assessment and formulation • The treatment

The models

The primary events in obsessive-compulsive disorder (OCD) are the obsessions, which can be defined as 'persistent thoughts, impulses, or images that are experienced as intrusive or inappropriate' (Wells, 1997, p. 236). The behavioural response to the obsession is the compulsion, which is seen as an attempt to *'neutralise'* the obsessional thoughts in some way. It is important to remember that OCD sufferers use a wide variety of neutralising compulsions. Some may be *overt* and clearly apparent to the onlooker, such as repeated washing of hands in those with obsessions with a theme of contamination. However, others will be much more *covert*. For example, many patients have counting rituals where they count in their head as a compulsive behaviour in response to an obsessive thought. This may not be apparent to an onlooker. If these covert behaviours are missed, the therapy is less likely to be successful!

A key finding has been that intrusive, obsessive-type thoughts are much *more common than previously thought*. Salkovskis and Kirk (1997) found that nine in ten of the general population report having experienced them at some time. One way in which OCD sufferers appear to differ from other people who experience intrusive thoughts is that the same type of thoughts distress them more (cause more *anxiety*). That is, it is not the thoughts themselves that dictate the response, but the individual's *evaluation of them* (van Oppen and Arntz, 1994; Salkovskis and Kirk, 1997). Because of this, OCD has been viewed by some as a 'phobia of intrusive thoughts' (Leahy and Holland, 2000). Some interpret these thoughts as evidence that the thoughts could cause the individual to 'act in an out of control way'. One of the author's patients had the intrusive thought that she would take her clothes off and run down the church aisle 'amok'. She interpreted the presence of these repeated thoughts as evidence that it could actually happen. This is an example of what has been termed *'thought–action fusion'* (TAF) (Rachman and Shafran, 1999), where the person believes that having the thought means that the event has happened or will be more likely to happen in the future. Therefore, having the thought leads to anxiety, which the client attempts to 'neutralise' or get rid of, by carrying out the act of the compulsion. In fact, there are two forms of TAF. The example given above concerns *probability* – thinking a thought increases the chance of a related event actually occurring in real life. The second form of TAF relates to the occasions when people have morally unacceptable or shameful intrusive obsessive thoughts. They view having these thoughts as morally equivalent to actually caring out the shameful acts. For example, some patients may have obsessive thoughts about wanting to harm a relative (despite liking the relative). They may carry out a compulsion to neutralise that 'awful thought'. It is obviously important to carry out a very detailed assessment in such cases that the patient does not truly wish harm on the person and does not in fact gain some satisfaction or gain from having these thoughts. These two forms of TAF have been described as *'perceived probability TAF'* and *'moral TAF'* (Rachman and Shafran, 1999).

Beliefs about TAF are only one of a number of *'processing errors'* that OCD sufferers make in their faulty interpretation of their obsessive thoughts. Another common error is a general overestimation of danger, frequently linked to a *lack of understanding of risk* or probability (Foa and Kozak, 1986). They overestimate the risk that a negative event will occur, e.g. of running a pedestrian down while driving through town, and they also frequently overestimate the risk that they will be held responsible and suffer reprisals should that negative event occur (Salkovskis and Kirk, 1997).

OCD sufferers use a number of strategies that have the effect of making the situation worse:

- attempts to *'neutralise'* the obsessive thoughts by carrying out behaviours (compulsions) related to the obsessive thought. For example, people who have intrusive thoughts about dirt may wash their hands. They learn that in the short-term carrying out these actions does succeed in reducing their anxiety and distress, and therefore over time they may carry out the compulsion more and more with reduced resistance (*operant conditioning*). Over time the distress of the obsessive thoughts causes the sufferer to repeat the actions more and more often in an increasing variety of ways, so that they develop a 'repertoire' of compulsions
- *thought suppression*: this is actively avoiding the obsessive thoughts by pushing them away. In common with the flashbacks encountered in PTSD, this appears to actively promote the persistence and frequency over time of the intrusive thoughts (Wegner, 1989; Trinder and Salkovskis 1994)
- *avoidance*: frequently, OCD sufferers simply avoid those places and situations that seem to precipitate their obsessive thoughts. Those with obsessive thoughts about the possibility of hurting others may stop driving. As the perceived relief of not experiencing the anxiety-inducing obsessive thoughts is linked in the sufferer's mind with having avoided the situation (another form of *operant conditioning*), so then the patient uses avoidance more and more
- *attention on thinking*: because of the fear of their obsessional thoughts, some OCD sufferers consciously monitor their own thoughts for obsessional themes (Wells, 1997). This monitoring behaviour may trigger more obsessional thoughts in the first place and certainly makes it more likely in the future that the patient will detect unwanted thoughts (Wells, 1997).

Assessment and formulation

The following information will normally be sought regarding OCD:

- what are the *predominant obsessive thoughts* endured by the client?
- what is the client's *usual strategy for coping* with the intrusive obsessional thoughts? Do they try and *'neutralise'* their obsessive thoughts (or more accurately the anxiety caused by the obsessional thought) with compulsive behaviours? If so, are these activities *overt*, or does the client undertake more subtle *covert* mental 'neutralising' activities?
- does the client *resist* thinking about their obsessive thoughts by trying to push them out of consciousness, and do they try and resist carrying out the compulsions?
- do they try to reduce the likelihood of having obsessional thoughts by *avoiding circumstances* that might precipitate them in the first place?
- what does the client fear would happen if they did not undertake these neutralising activities – the *feared consequence*? What evidence do they hold for this?
- as always, are there any *modifiers* – i.e. what makes the frequency and intensity of the obsessive thoughts worse and what makes them better? Under what conditions is the client more or less likely to respond to the thoughts by carrying out rituals? In particular ask about the influence of stress
- are there any *co-morbid* mental health problems – e.g. depression, anxiety, and substance misuse?
- what have been the *consequences of the OCD* on the sufferer's life? In particular, are they still able to work?
- finally, in view of the fact that OCD does tend to be a *chronically remitting disorder*, what has brought the client for treatment at this present time?

Example

Jamie is 32 and lives with his mother and younger brother. The only obsessive thought that Jamie could identify was that he would 'get ill and even die from an infection'. He thought that other people's germs would be especially dangerous and that they would be likely to cause 'septicaemia' (his word!) if they got anywhere near a skin wound. He constantly worries that the toilet is too close to the bath. He accepted that these thoughts were 'over the top', but 'had upsetting thoughts about germs all day', so has increasingly just 'given in to the urge' to clean. He does not even try to resist the thoughts now, but simply stays in the flat all day to avoid germs. He routinely gets up after everyone else has left the house in order that he can start his complex regime of cleaning the whole bathroom with bleach. He then showers three times, using a separate clean towel between each shower. At lunchtime he has a further shower and another before going to bed. Between each shower he repeats the rituals of cleaning the bathroom with bleach. He has carried out this pattern of cleaning and showering for 13 years, but 'normally' only showers twice in the morning and sometimes not at all after that. Jamie's father died unexpectedly one year ago. This had been a huge loss to Jamie who was tearful when discussing this.

A *formulation* integrating the above information could be:

This man presents with obsessional thoughts with a theme of contamination. To some degree he accepts that his concerns are excessive, but he also appears to be truly overestimating risk, possibly as a consequence of a lack of knowledge. He tries to cope with his obsessive thoughts by carrying out a number of cleaning compulsions. His resistance to these compulsions has reduced over time and is now minimal. His symptoms are aggravated by stress in the home, and generally have worsened since the death of his father one year ago. There are no clear alleviating factors. Apart from carrying out his compulsive cleaning, his predominant coping strategy has been to use avoidance. He avoids all social contacts outside of his family and is now housebound as a consequence of his attempts to avoid 'germs'. His avoidance prevents exposure to situations that would otherwise help to counter his beliefs of risk, and because the avoidance takes away the anxiety it is reinforced over time through operant conditioning. His avoidance has increased to the point where it causes significant functional impairment, including an inability to remain in employment.

The treatment

Note that clients who are severely depressed or who respond to their distress by using illicit substances need to address these before treating the OCD.

- The CBT approach to OCD usually involves some *psycho-education* about the disorder. This will include discussion about the large proportion of the population that experience obsessive-type thoughts, and the fact that they are not dangerous. The negative effects of avoidance and thought suppression are also normally addressed. The latter can be further illustrated with the use of the '*pink polar bear experiment*'. The therapist asks the client to think of anything but a pink polar bear for 30 seconds or a minute. The patient finds that they cannot totally prevent thoughts about pink polar bears from intrusively entering their mind. This illustrates the fact that active thought suppression is an ineffective way of preventing obsessional thoughts from entering consciousness – and can even make matters worse.
- *Exposure and response prevention* (ERP) remains the most important element of the cognitive behavioural approach to OCD. In common with other disorders described in this book, the required exposure can be in the form of both '*imaginal exposure*' and '*in vivo exposure*'. Where OCD is different from disorders requiring simple exposure is that the *exposure must be linked with response prevention*. Repeated exposure works to reduce the client's anxiety when they experience the intrusive obsessive thoughts, via a number of mechanisms. Firstly, exposure helps to change the belief that thoughts are powerful and dangerous by proving that simply thinking a distressing thought does not lead to a catastrophic outcome (reduces belief in TAF). Secondly, when the client allows him or herself to experience the obsessional thoughts over and over again without a

negative outcome, they *habituate* to them. Thirdly, if they successfully stop themselves from carrying out the compulsions (the response prevention), then they learn that the feared outcome will not be the result of failing to carry out that behaviour. The client is asked to construct a *hierarchy of obsessional thoughts*. This is simply a list of all the experienced obsessive thoughts graded by the amount of distress they cause. The client then relays back to the therapist in as much detail as possible the content of these obsessional thoughts and the catastrophic feared consequences starting with less distressing ones and eventually working up to the most distressing thoughts. *Where the client has compulsions these are stopped (the response prevention) and the client stays with and habituates to the underlying obsessional thoughts.* Generally the client moves up the hierarchy so that the most difficult obsessional thoughts/compulsions are tackled last.

- *Where there are no compulsions but only obsessional thoughts*, then these thoughts are normally audio-taped and the client is instructed to listen to their taped accounts over and over in a 'taped loop' at home, in order to maximise habituation.
- Where *actual situations are avoided* due to their association with the obsessional thoughts, then an in vivo exposure approach is taken in exactly the same way as described in Chapter 9. However, care must be taken to resist carrying out the neutralising compulsions concurrent with the exposure.
- *Beliefs about catastrophe and overestimation of danger* can be challenged using standard cognitive techniques such as the use of dysfunctional thought records. In particular the probability of any event occurring can be assessed by breaking the end event down into all the component events and asking the client what the probability of each of the component events occurring would be (van Oppen and Arntz, 1994). The risk of each component event occurring is multiplied together to give an overall estimation of risk as discussed in Chapter 10. In Jamie's case the chance that a dangerous bacteria was present in the environment may be one in forty, the chance that he would have an open skin wound may be one in ten, the chance the bacteria would land in the wound may also be one in ten and the chance that his body would not be capable of fighting the bacteria may be one in a hundred. Multiplying all of these probabilities together would mean that he had a one in 400000 chance of contracting a fatal infection after contact with friends!
- *Beliefs about responsibility and thought–action fusion* should also be addressed using the same standard cognitive strategies, such as dysfunctional thought records and psycho-education. For example, a patient with distress at having intrusive thoughts about dropping her baby could be treated using a thought record. A key underlying belief may be: 'having the thought of dropping my baby means I'm evil'. An investigation into the patient's intent, wishes and controllability of her thoughts might help to reduce the degree of belief in this thought and may reduce the chances of them engaging in subsequent 'neutralising' compulsive behaviours or avoidance. As stated before, it is obviously important to clearly assess that there is actually no significant risk – i.e. that the person in this case does not actually want to drop the baby!

Jamie agreed somewhat reluctantly to try CBT with a trainee, for his symptoms of OCD. The trainee had supervision with an experienced therapist. The therapy began with the trainee 'normalising' intrusive thoughts by explaining that they are common and not dangerous in themselves. Jamie was helped to compile both a hierarchy of feared obsessional thoughts and a hierarchy of avoided situations. Jamie agreed to try and postpone his showers by having a 20 minute 'break' between his three morning showers. The therapist aimed to use this to illustrate that there would not be catastrophic outcomes from stopping or postponing the compulsions. He then planned to carry out cognitive work looking at the true risk of getting an infection from 'germs in the bathroom'. Unfortunately, when the therapist later asked Jamie whether he had successfully postponed his showering, he had not. The supervisor suggested that the trainee 'go back to basics' and consider the underlying diagnosis. It became clear that Jamie was depressed in the moderate range (BDI-II score of 26). An action plan was agreed that Jamie should be prescribed an SSRI antidepressant medication by his GP. The trainee therapist agreed to review Jamie six weeks later. At this follow-up Jamie was significantly brighter. He was once again only showering twice in the morning (and bleaching once). Jamie no longer considered his OCD symptoms a significant problem – 'I've always been like that' – but requested CBT sessions with the trainee for depression and to look at how to cope with the loss of his father.

MAIN POINTS

- Compulsions can be overt or covert. All compulsions need to be carefully identified to allow habituation to anxiety caused by the obsessive thoughts to occur.
- Intrusive thoughts are far more common in the general population than previously known. OCD can therefore be considered to relate more to how individuals respond to these thoughts rather than to whether they have them or not.
- An inaccurate estimation of probability and beliefs about 'thought–action fusion' also helps to maintain the disorder along with thought suppression, avoidance of the circumstances that precipitate the thoughts, and the monitoring (or scanning) of thoughts for obsessional themes.
- A vital component of treatment is 'exposure and response prevention' (ERP). In common with other exposure treatments, a hierarchy is constructed and the patient is exposed (or exposes themselves) to more distressing obsessive thoughts.
- Exposure to audio-taped obsessional thoughts spoken out loud, over and over on a 'taped loop', is a major way of achieving exposure to obsessive thoughts where there are no compulsions.
- Psycho-education about the nature and frequency of obsessional thoughts within the general population (normalisation) plays an important role in treatment, as does education about risk and probabilities, and the concept of 'thought–action fusion'.

Further reading

- Leahy RL and Holland SJ (2000) *Treatment Plans and Interventions for Depression and Anxiety Disorders*. New York: Guilford Press.
- Rachman S (2003) *The treatment of obsessions*. Oxford: Oxford University Press.
- Salkovskis PM and Kirk J (1997) Obsessive-compulsive disorder. In: Clark DM and Fairburn CG (eds) *Science and Practice of Cognitive Behaviour Therapy*. Oxford: Oxford University Press, pp. 179–208.

Chapter 12

Cognitive behavioural therapy applied to post-traumatic stress disorder

The models • Assessment and formulation • The treatment

The models

The general theme of most models of PTSD is that severe trauma *overwhelms* the individual with information that is difficult to process. Therefore, PTSD represents a state of functioning where information relating to an event remains *unprocessed* (Rachman, 1980). It is proposed that this applies to raw material unprocessed in memory and also to the *personal meaning* (appraisal) ascribed to what has happened (Ehlers and Clark, 2000). It is proposed that after a trauma we try and re-process this information in order to integrate our experiences, something referred to as a *'completion tendency'* (Horowitz, 1986). We therefore re-experience unprocessed material from memory, which comes back as flashbacks, nightmares and possibly in ruminative thoughts. The mind is *re-presenting the information* in order that it can be properly integrated.

Sensations that the individual experienced at the time of the trauma can become associated with the distress of the trauma (Mowrer, 1960). For example, patients who have suffered a road traffic accident (RTA) can become anxious when confronted with the smell of spilled oil. Prior to the RTA the smell of oil would not have elicited anxiety. The process that is occurring here is *classical conditioning*. There is also a process of *generalisation*, whereby not only the original sensation evokes an emotional response, but also similar sensations. Therefore, the RTA patient may develop anxiety and indeed may experience disabling flashbacks when confronted with the smell of oil, petrol, or a variety of similar smells such as cleaning materials. The individual, not surprisingly, tries to avoid these *'conditioned stimuli'*, with the effect that in the short term the level of experienced anxiety (and flashbacks) is lowered. Unfortunately, because the individual learns that their anxiety can be reduced by *avoidance*, this increasingly becomes a part of their strategy of coping. It is this avoidance of both real situations and distressing thoughts that acts to maintain both the anxiety and the flashbacks (Mowrer, 1960; Ehlers and Clark, 2000). Avoidance tends to increase anxiety in the longer term, as patients never have the chance to learn that the feared situation is not as dangerous as they presume. As the relief of not experiencing the anxiety or flashbacks is linked in the sufferer's mind with having avoided the situation (*operant conditioning*), the patient uses avoidance more and more (Mowrer,

1960). A similar process occurs when PTSD sufferers try and avoid their intrusive thoughts and flashbacks. One of the most common methods of trying to cope with them is to actively avoid them by pushing them away, a behaviour known as *'thought suppression'*. There is evidence that this merely acts to promote their persistence and frequency over time (Trinder and Salkovskis, 1994).

Janoff-Bulman (1992) describes how sometimes the experiences involved in trauma are so extreme that they *'shatter' pre-existing beliefs and assumptions* that the client holds about them, other people and the world around them. This can be compounded by the material losses experienced.

Finally, *'complex trauma'* or 'complex PTSD' refers to multiple traumas, previous traumas having probably made a PTSD response to a subsequent trauma more likely. The presentation is made more complex because of the interaction of the previous events, particularly when they have impacted on the patient's personality development. Commonly it is seen in people who have survived traumas such as abuse in childhood, which has placed them at increased risk of responding negatively to traumas with a similar theme later in life.

Assessment and formulation

The following information needs to be sought in relation to PTSD:

- Are there major symptoms of PTSD present? PTSD as described in DSM-IV comprises three main symptom areas. These are: *re-experiencing symptoms*, (including 'flashbacks' and nightmares), *increased arousal*, (including sleep disturbance and an increased 'startle response'), and finally *avoidance* (not only of places they associate with the trauma, but also of thinking about the events)
- As always, are there any *modifiers* – that is what makes the symptoms worse and what makes them better?
- A thorough assessment of the *events of the trauma* itself: in particular ask what it was about the trauma that was the most difficult aspect for the patient, and why
- What is the patient's appraisal of their activity within the trauma period? Do they have *guilt or shame*, and do they view themselves/others/the world differently now?
- Are there *co-morbid mental health problems* – particularly depression, anxiety and panic, substance abuse and hallucinations? There may be *personality change*, best assessed by a corroborative history from a friend or relative who knew the patient both before and after the trauma
- What coping strategies are used? Do they use *avoidance* and *safety behaviours*?
- What have been the effects of the trauma and PTSD on the sufferer's life, e.g. have they isolated themselves from others or reduced their activity levels?
- Are there any *previous traumas* that may have made the patient at increased risk of responding negatively to the current 'index trauma'?
- Finally, are there any circumstances such as *uncertain asylum status* or a forthcoming *court case* that may be influencing the presentation or the history given?

Example

Murat is a 51-year-old man who survived a devastating earthquake in Iran and who has since been granted asylum status in the UK. He suffers from severe flashbacks that are vivid in his mind as if he were 'experiencing the earthquake all over again'. The flashbacks are at their worst at night when it is quiet. Nothing makes them better. He has a vivid 'image' of his nephew dying after being hit with masonry. He utterly blames himself for his nephew's death in that he witnessed the falling masonry and believes he 'could have pushed him out of the way'. Murat physically 'jumps at anything'. He also avoids going into the city centre, and he intermittently scans the sides of high buildings for dangerous masonry. Life holds little enjoyment for him; he feels depressed and lethargic and he avoids contact with others. He sleeps through the day. He is unable to sleep at night due to the flashbacks. He has not used drugs or alcohol to excess, does not have a prior history of trauma, and did not have low mood or any of the above symptoms prior to the earthquake. Both Murat and his wife described how he had changed – previously he had been a very 'sociable man' who had worked in Iran as a panel beater.

A *formulation* could include:

This man presents with all three main symptom areas of PTSD. Namely, he suffers from severe re-experiencing of symptoms, he has increased arousal in the form of sleep problems and increased startle response, and he avoids thinking about the trauma (cognitive avoidance) as well as avoiding situations that have become associated with the trauma such as high buildings. He also has symptoms of a depressive episode. He is disabled by his flashbacks, which are aggravated by being alone at night. His appraisal of the trauma event is that he failed to save a relative's life. This has left him with strong feelings of shame and associated questions about his own self-worth. His predominant coping strategy has been to use avoidance. He actively attempts not to think about what happened, which probably results in an increased chance that thoughts will intrude upon his consciousness. He has socially isolated himself from those people who would previously have provided protective support. This was a man whose work and social contacts were previously an important part of his life and probably helped him to define his own identity. The loss of these is a further maintaining factor for his depressed mood and his belief that he is worthless.

The treatment

- *Psycho-education* forms a part of the CBT approach to PTSD. 'Normalising' the symptoms of PTSD as a disorder and not as evidence of characterological weakness or evidence that the patient is 'going mad' is an important part of treatment.

- *Exposure forms the mainstay of the current CBT approach to PTSD.* This can be in the form of both 'imaginal exposure' and 'in vivo exposure'.
- In *imaginal exposure* the client is asked to construct a *hierarchy* of the most *distressing memories* of the traumatic events. Normally these will correspond to the content of the flashbacks. The client then imagines and relays back to the therapist in as much detail as possible the content of the memories, starting with less distressing ones and eventually working onto the most distressing memories. On recounting the memories the client is exposed to them, and on repeated exposure becomes *habituated* to them. To maximise the exposure, the recounting is normally audio-taped, and the client is instructed to listen to their taped accounts at home. Occasionally where the amount of distress caused is very high, this is only done within the session.
- If there are specific *feared situations* – the site of a disaster or places that have become associated with the trauma through conditioning – then the client can become less fearful and avoidant of them through *in vivo exposure*. Once again the client constructs a hierarchy of feared situations. They are slowly exposed to them and habituate to situations progressively higher up the hierarchy.
- Teaching *anxiety-management techniques* such as abdominal breathing and progressive muscular relaxation may be needed to allow some clients to continue with the exposure tasks.
- *Eye movement desensitisation and reprocessing* (EMDR) (Shapiro, 1995) can be used. This is generally a two-stage process. The client is initially asked to reflect back and so begins to *process* the traumatic image. At this stage the imagery is still combined with associated negative thoughts – for example, thinking about a car accident whilst thinking: 'It was my fault, I'm so stupid'. The second step may be to install a new more positive cognition such as: 'I had a car accident – they occur commonly' and to pair this new interpretation with the initial imagery. Here the client is asked to focus on the unpleasant images and thoughts relating to the traumatic event and then to imagine alternative appraisals of what actually happened. The therapist elicits *rapid lateral eye movements* in the client, by asking them to focus on the therapist's finger that tracks from side to side in front of the client's face (other techniques are also used with the same aim). The patient does not need to discuss the content of their re-experiencing of past events with the therapist, and for this reason some very traumatised clients cope better with EMDR than with classic in-session exposure, which requires the client to speak their thoughts out loud. It is not clear how EMDR exerts its effects, but exposure probably plays a part.
- *Key unhelpful beliefs and assumptions* about the trauma and the patient's response to it can also be addressed. For example, if the client unreasonably believes that their actions were to blame for negative outcomes, then this can be investigated using techniques such as thought records.

> Murat's symptoms were 'normalised' by the therapist, and it was then agreed that the flashbacks would be addressed using imaginal exposure. An exposure hierarchy was constructed – thoughts about his nephew's death were the most distressing. In time Murat was able to tolerate exposure outside the session; this resulted in habituation – a reduction in his subjective levels of

distress. It also allowed him to be able to discuss his story with his friend who, together with the therapist, encouraged Murat to question whether the death of his nephew had really been his fault. His belief changed, and his associated feelings of shame reduced. He agreed to increase activity levels. Social isolation was addressed by his enrolment in English classes and joining a Farsi social club. His mood was seen to improve on BDI ratings. After four graded in vivo exposure sessions he was able to walk to the most built-up areas of the city and had stopped scanning for falling masonry (he dropped his safety behaviour). Finally, he was able to take part-time employment, which further increased his social contacts and further eroded his belief that he was worthless.

MAIN POINTS

- People's response to trauma varies – PTSD is only one response, a depressive reaction may be another.
- Avoidance of stimuli that remind the patient of the trauma acts to maintain PTSD though operant conditioning.
- Pre-existing beliefs and assumptions about the world can be shattered by a traumatic event.
- 'Complex trauma' or 'complex PTSD' refers to multiple traumas, previous traumas having probably made a PTSD response to a subsequent trauma more likely.
- A corroborative history from someone who knew the patient before the traumatic event can be essential because of potential personality change and changes in the way that people relate to others after a trauma.
- Treatment is exposure based: both imaginal exposure (to the events of the trauma to encourage cognitive processing), and exposure in vivo (to allow habituation to avoided situations associated with the trauma).
- Eye-movement desensitisation and reprocessing (EMDR) is used to treat PTSD. It assists with re-processing the trauma memories, although the exact mechanism of action is debated.

Further reading

- Ehlers A and Clark DM (2000) A cognitive model of persistent posttraumatic stress disorder. *Behaviour Research and Therapy* **38**: 319–45.
- Shapiro F (1995) *Eye Movement Desensitisation and Reprocessing: basic principles, protocols and procedures.* New York: Guilford.

Chapter 13

Cognitive behavioural therapy applied to anorexia nervosa and bulimia nervosa

The models • Assessment and formulation • The treatment

The models

There is significant overlap between anorexia nervosa (AN) and bulimia nervosa (BN) in terms of symptoms and the models that describe the factors that maintain the disorders. Furthermore, those suffering from one disorder have an increased chance of developing the other disorder later in life (Vitousek, 1996).

Vitousek proposes that both bulimia and anorexia are maintained by character-istic *rigid and extreme assumptions about body shape and weight* that are strongly influenced by the culture in which the patient lives. Examples of such rules are: 'fat people are worth less than thin people' and: 'fat people are lazy'. They are also likely to have schemas relating to themselves as worthless or defective. People with both AN and BN are particularly likely to have *perfectionistic* personality traits and to use dichotomous thinking (*'all or nothing' thinking*) (Fairburn, 1997). They often hold *rigid and extreme beliefs* in the area of eating patterns and weight. For example, many believe that if they eat a very small amount of a fattening food they will gain weight. This often leads to extreme corresponding *'all or nothing' behaviours*, such as severely restricting food intake for long periods and avoiding certain 'bad' foods completely.

A leading *model of bulimia* (Fairburn, 1997) proposes that the key maintaining factor is the tendency to judge self-worth in terms of weight or shape. This causes individuals to restrict their food intake in order that they might attain that weight or shape. In BN, the resulting psychological and physiological effects of restricting food intake as well as dichotomous thinking ('now I've had one chocolate I might as well just eat them all'), result in episodes of *binge eating* (Fairburn, 1997). In the short term, bingeing allows them to feel better, for example, by alleviating feelings of depression. The bingeing is therefore 'positively reinforced' (operant condition-ing). However, after feeling better from bingeing, the patient experiences *guilt* at violating their rules about food intake. This results in the use of *reversing behaviours* to undo the effects of overeating, including self-induced vomiting or laxative use as well as *restricting food intake* in between episodes of bingeing. These help to *maintain the focus* of the bulimic's thoughts on shape, weight and self-worth, and therefore increase the chance of engaging in future bingeing (Fairburn, 1997). Restricting food intake by physiological means appears to increase the likelihood of subsequent bingeing behaviours (Polivy and Herman, 1995).

Self-control is particularly important in *models of anorexia nervosa*. Control over *eating and weight* are used by anorexics as pointers of overall 'self-control' – and, by extension, of *self-worth* (Fairburn *et al*, 1999). Vitousek (Vitousek, 1996) reasons that when anorexics are successful in restricting their diet, they feel better about themselves. This therefore *positively reinforces* the restricting behaviour (operant conditioning). Being able to avoid the fear of being fat also *negatively reinforces* the behaviours. Their underlying schemas regarding shape, weight and self-worth cause them to *interpret day-to-day events in a biased way*. For example, a failed interview may be interpreted as being down to: 'looking too fat'. This biased thinking further reinforces the anorexic behaviours of restricting food intake etc. Finally, the *effects of starvation* may serve to worsen the very concrete, dichotomous thinking style. The anorexic also frequently isolates him- or herself and attempts to *gain back a sense of control* in the way they know best – to further restrict food intake (Vitousek, 1996).

Assessment and formulation

The following information needs to be sought in relation to AN and BN:

- the current weight and height and a calculated *body mass index* (BMI)
- engagement in *weight-restriction behaviours* designed to induce weight loss or minimise weight gain, such as excessive exercise, calorie restriction, laxative or diuretic use, and self-induced vomiting
- evidence of *episodes of overeating* over short periods. It is best to document carefully a typical episode of overeating. How do emotional changes influence what happens? For example, does low mood precipitate the overeating, and is the mood alleviated by doing so?
- is the client particularly afraid of being fat? They may have a perceived '*ideal weight*' that may be both exact and low
- is there a *distorted body image* – that is does the patient believe they are fat when they are obviously not?
- as always, are there any *modifiers* of the symptoms, e.g. what seems to precipitate and exacerbate bulimic episode frequency, what makes the patient's weight rise and fall?
- what is the least and the most that the patient has weighed?
- what has the client used to *try and cope* with their symptoms, such as avoidance of friendships, of relationships, or of simply eating in front of others?
- what have been the *consequences* of their symptoms in terms of family, social, psychological, and physical effects?
- what are the patient's *schemas* of himself or herself? What are the predominant fears and *assumptions* driving the disorder? Is there evidence of characteristic *cognitive distortions*, in particular 'all or nothing' thinking?
- what is the patient's attitude towards their symptoms? Is the patient *motivated to change*? What are the perceived benefits and fears of change?

- are there any *co-morbid mental health problems* – particularly OCD, depression or personality problems?

Example

Ami is a 17-year-old student. Her BMI is just over 20 (normal), and she has never weighed significantly more or less than this. Her 'perfect' weight is only 4 lb less than her current weight. She is continuing to menstruate and there is no evidence of other mental health conditions. She is currently taking her first year university examinations. Her bingeing has got worse in the last few weeks and it also did during her 'AS' levels in school. She comes home every night and immediately binges on large volumes of carbohydrate-rich food. Immediately afterwards she feels 'relieved', but then feels 'terror' that she is going to put on weight. Without exception she makes herself vomit. She is ashamed that she does this and is also ashamed that she believes herself to be overweight. She copes with her shame by avoiding her classmates. She was explicit in her view that 'thin women are more worthy', citing a number of successful actresses as examples. She hopes to lose the weight after the exams, and expects to look 'acceptable' to her classmates at that point. To that end she spends most evenings either revising or in the gym. She also compares 'how bad' she looks relative to the other women in the gym and feels ashamed. At times this results in Ami having to leave the gym pre-maturely, and has resulted in her engaging in overeating to alleviate her 'bad feelings'.

A *formulation* could include:

Ami presents with behaviours that form part of the diagnosis of bulimia nervosa including episodes of overeating, self-induced vomiting, and excessive exercise. These behaviours are positively reinforced in that they alleviate the stress that Ami feels, albeit only momentarily. After the immediate relief, however, they cause Ami to be distressed that she has broken her strict 'eating rules' and that they have placed her at risk of gaining weight. She therefore attempts to quickly reverse the effects of overeating using self-induced vomiting. Ami's behaviour and thoughts are driven by her assumption that 'thin women are more worthy'. She also shows 'all or nothing' thinking, in that she expects only 4 lb weight loss would make her 'socially acceptable', whereas she is 'not socially acceptable at her current weight'. She therefore avoids talking to her classmates, expecting that they will shun her. Ami frequently compares her body shape with that of other women, a behaviour which further maintains her preoccupation with body shape and food intake. The body shape comparisons and avoidance of social contact add to the overall distress that Ami feels. This makes it more likely that she will overeat as a means of trying to reduce her distress, thus creating a vicious circle. Stress is a key modifier, particularly during periods of examinations, that serves to further maintain the above vicious circle.

The treatment

In general, CBT for anorexia typically lasts for 1–2 years. CBT for bulimia is much shorter (10–20 sessions), although some cases do need longer. AN clients need longer treatments due to the emphasis on schema change, motivational issues and the worse prognosis. The approach to eating disorders generally includes:

- *motivation to change*: before starting treatment for AN it should be explained to the client that if they go below a certain weight (measured as a BMI index), then they will require more intensive treatment – normally day hospital or inpatient status for re-feeding. Once a degree of motivation has been secured, a *target weight* is agreed upon. This is normally about 90% of the expected BMI. Weighing usually occurs at the beginning of the session of the AN client. BN clients whose weight is not a concern usually self-weigh outside of the sessions. Initial sessions tend to have an emphasis on fostering the therapeutic relationship as well as addressing motivational issues
- *psycho-education*: this forms an important part of the treatment of both AN and BN (Garner, 1997). For example, AN clients are told about the features of starvation and that they are akin to the features witnessed by anorexia sufferers. These include a preoccupation with food, binge eating, depression, and a range of physical problems such parasthesia and oedema (Garner, 1997). In BN the effects of the purging such as biochemical disturbance and the loss of tooth enamel with self-induced vomiting are usually explored
- *self-monitoring*: this is an essential part of CBT throughout the treatment of both AN and BN. It can take the form of diaries that show changes in food intake, laxative use, exercise and weight as appropriate. The thoughts that precede the behaviours are particularly useful to gather and challenge using DTRs as described in Chapter 6. An example may be to challenge the thought 'I've lost control of my eating today' by looking at the supporting and non-supporting evidence to assess the validity of the automatic thought
- *experimentation with behaviour change*: once the patient has begun to successfully monitor their behaviours, weight and thoughts, then the effects of experimenting with behavioural change can progress. Importantly, clients find that the *urge to binge or vomit does not continue to increase* if they continue to resist carrying out that behaviour beyond a certain time. The urge normally increases to a point and then begins to dissipate
- *meal planning*: this involves making decisions about what is going to be eaten in advance. There needs to be clear monitoring of the degree of adherence and the effects of the intervention. The four main elements of meal planning advocated by Garner *et al* (1997) are:
  - *mechanical eating* – eating in a mechanical way takes some of the decision making out of eating
  - *spacing eating* – having spaced-out, pre-set times for eating (normally 3 meals and 1–2 snacks daily) reduces cravings for food, and re-introduces control in eating
  - *increasing the quantity of food* – the calorific content of food to be consumed can be pre-set. This will be particularly important for AN patients

- *broadening the range of food* – previously avoided 'bad' foods should be re-introduced in small amounts. For example in BN, foods normally only eaten in binges should be gradually introduced as part of the non-binge diet
- *changing underlying assumptions and schemas*: this is a major component of the CBT approach to eating disorders, particularly for those patients who clearly link self-worth and weight
- *relapse prevention*: a relapse into one episode of bingeing may be interpreted as 'all is lost – I'm back to square one' (dichotomous thinking). Relapses should be reframed as opportunities to further learn and practise interventions (Garner 1997).

As homework Ami monitored her thoughts and behaviours, including her bingeing and vomiting. The diary confirmed typical 'all or nothing' thinking at a number of points. This included the point when she had eaten a small amount of refined carbohydrate when she believed she had broken her rule of not eating that sort of food so: 'it didn't matter any more'. Ami learnt about the negative effects of dieting and self-induced vomiting. Eventually, she agreed to experiment with two changes. One was to stop both bingeing and vomiting for a day; the second was to reintroduce the forbidden food of chocolate into her diet in small amounts. She was successful at the latter task, but she could not resist the urge to binge. The therapist suggested that Ami was hungry on returning home, and that she should plan to eat a larger lunch, and maybe pre-prepare a nutritious snack for her return home. This was a huge success – she ate a significantly larger lunch (pre-prepared by Ami the night before), and also had some vegetable soup waiting at home to be re-heated on her arrival. She was relieved that her weight did not rise despite her changes. Ami explored the validity of the assumption: 'thin women are more worthy', by asking the views of a number of trusted female friends (variety of ages). She also looked at a number of other 'successful women' who were in the news but who were not thin. She had previously 'discounted these people – somehow'.

MAIN POINTS

- Clients with BN and AN frequently hold rigid and extreme assumptions about weight and body shape. They also commonly have perfectionistic personality traits and engage in dichotomous ('all or nothing') thinking.
- BN and AN clients also engage in 'all or nothing' behaviours, such as completely avoiding certain 'bad' foods.
- Fairburn's model of BN proposes that sufferers judge their own self-worth by their shape or their weight. Binge eating is a consequence of 'all or nothing' thinking and food restriction. Bingeing is also reinforced (operant conditioning) by the alleviation of distress that it can give in the short term.
- 'Reversing behaviours' such as food restriction maintain the focus of thoughts on food and eating.

- Self-control (and the perceived negative implications on self-worth of not having it!) is a key maintaining factor in AN.
- The effects of starvation can be to cause impaired concentration, and more extreme dichotomous thinking, which can lead to a worsening clinical state in a vicious circle.
- Due to risk, and the greater emphasis on schema-change, CBT for AN usually lasts much longer than CBT for BN.
- Psycho-education plays a major role in CBT for both disorders, as does the experimentation with (or 'prescription of') new eating habits, such as eating in a 'spaced out' and 'mechanical' fashion.

Further reading

- Fairburn CG, Shafran R and Cooper Z (1999) A cognitive–behavioural theory of anorexia nervosa. *Behaviour Research and Therapy* **37**: 1–13.
- Vitousek K (1996) The current status of cognitive-behavioural models of anorexia nervosa and bulimia nervosa. In: Salkovskis PM (ed) *Frontiers of Cognitive Therapy*. New York: Guilford Press, pp. 383–418.

Chapter 14

Cognitive behavioural therapy applied to hallucinations and delusions

The models • Assessment and formulation • The treatment

The models

Fundamental principles behind CBT for psychosis are that:

- there is more of a *continuum between delusional and non-delusional thinking* and *between hallucinations and normal experiences* than previously considered. Therefore, we see members of the general public who hold beliefs despite clear evidence to the contrary. Likewise, the number of people in the community who hear voices is now known to be far greater than once thought (Tien, 1992)
- the *content of both hallucinations and delusions can often be understood* within the 'interpersonal context of a person's life' (Kingdon and Turkington, 1994). Therefore, clients with a history of abuse may develop paranoid beliefs with a theme corresponding to past events, and clients with a strong faith may develop delusions with a prominent religious content.

These principles mark a significant departure from traditional psychiatric teaching, which frequently viewed the content of delusions and hallucinations as fundamentally non-understandable.

In common with the way that cognitive biases maintain depression, similar mechanisms appear to play a role in maintaining delusions and hallucinations. The biases are those previously encountered in depression – 'all or nothing' thinking, selective abstraction, etc. In addition, clients with psychosis have a tendency to make *external and personal attributions for negative events* (Kinderman and Bentall, 1997). This means that they have a tendency to blame negative outcomes on the actions of others rather than on themselves, and they are overly inclined to see these actions as having been intentionally carried out specifically to harm them. Psychotic clients as a group have also been noted to possess *poor problem-solving skills* and to have a tendency to *jump to conclusions* when presented with only limited evidence (Garety and Hemsley, 1994).

A major behavioural maintaining factor is the use of *avoidance*. In a similar way that a socially phobic client avoids social situations, so psychotic clients avoid people or places that they perceive as threatening. They fail to realise that the place or person they avoid is not as threatening as they believe. This reinforces their belief in the threat, and encourages further avoidance.

Clients who develop hallucinations may be biologically *predisposed* to hearing their thoughts as voices or seeing them as images (Morrison and Haddock, 1997). In addition, both the way that the client *views* the voices and *what they then do* about them can function to maintain them. It has been proposed that the client's beliefs about the voices are more important in predicting the distress experienced and the behaviour towards the voices, than their objective content (Chadwick and Birchwood, 1994). Many clients view their voices as intrusive and threatening. Some use the evidence that they appear to know all about the client's past as evidence that the voices are extremely powerful. Their response is to believe what they say, or to do what the voices command – for fear of retribution should they not do so. This attitude of *helplessness* can result in depression or reduced compliance with medication. The distressed (or depressed) emotional state and the cessation of medication can both function to maintain the voices or maintain the client's distress towards the voices. Other behaviours, such as isolating themselves from others, perhaps from fear that the voices could make them harm others, further aggravates their sense of hopelessness and tendency to sit and ruminate upon the content and implications of the voices (Romme *et al*, 1992). This further maintains the voices. Because of the avoidance of those situations where their unhelpful beliefs about the voices could be put to the test, their beliefs are further maintained (Morrison, 1998). Clients who attempt to 'neutralise' their voices by resisting them, by talking back at them, also frequently have a resulting increase in their voice activity. Likewise, distraction does not work. Therefore, many clients find that that accepting their voices, learning not to have strong emotional reactions to what is being said, and not trying to resist or divert attention is effective in allowing the voices to settle (Romme *et al*, 1992).

Assessment and formulation

The following information needs to be sought regarding *delusional beliefs*:

- the *content* of the beliefs, and the extent to which they are '*mood congruent*'. This will help to discriminate between an affective diagnosis and other diagnoses such as an organic or schizophreniform illness
- what were the *events* around the time that they started? How have the delusion(s) developed over time?
- what are the *modifiers* – that is does anything seem to make the beliefs more or less intense/firmly held?
- are there any *benefits* for the patient in holding the delusion? For example, does a persecutory belief about the actions of a neighbour prevent the client from considering the persecutory behaviour that he himself may have directed towards this man in the past?
- is there *risk inherent* in holding the delusional belief(s), such as potential danger towards themselves or others? A full risk assessment would include whether the patient has ever acted on these delusions in the past, concurrent substance abuse and a history of other forensic issues
- what other *coping strategies* does the patient try to use – what effect do they have?

- how do the *delusions* relate to any hallucinatory experiences if these are present?
- finally, are there other *potential causes* of the delusions – e.g. illicit or prescribed drugs or alcohol problems?

For *hallucinations*, from a CBT perspective we are particularly interested to know the following:

- the *content of the hallucinations* in as much detail as possible. This will help to diagnose the underlying condition. In particular, are the voices mood congruent?
- when did the *hallucinations start*? How have the hallucinations developed over time?
- do they recognise the voice(s)? If so, is there *significance in the voice* that is heard, e.g. a previous abuser?
- *modifiers*: what makes the voices louder/quieter, and what makes them occur less often and more often? This may give clues to maintaining factors such as avoidance
- how are the *voices viewed* – as a friend or foe? Are they viewed as powerful?
- does the voice *command* the patient to do things? Can the client resist? What are they afraid would happen if they did resist or did not resist?
- what other *coping strategies* does the patient try to use, and what effect do they have?
- how do the voices relate to *delusions* if these are present?
- finally, are there other *potential causes* of the hallucinations – e.g. illicit or prescribed drugs or alcohol problems?

Example

Jeannie is a 29-year-old woman living with her mother. She has been diagnosed with schizophrenia. She hears one voice outside of her head, which speaks to her directly (in the second person). She does not recognise the voice and she does not have a name for it. The voice has been with Jeannie for about 7 years, since the time that she had chosen to leave her job (because she was being bullied). The voice seems to get worse when she is tired or stressed. She is unable to identify times when it is less prominent. The voice appears to use information about Jeannie's past, and Jeannie views this as evidence of how clever and powerful the voice is. Very occasionally the voice gives her commands such as: 'pick up the fork' or: 'pull her hair'. She has tended to comply with these unless the commands are dangerous. Her response to the voice is to: 'go quiet' and 'avoid others'. The voice had told her that her brother (who lived apart from the family) was 'evil'. It had not, however, told her to harm her brother. She consequently avoided her brother and when she heard about his failed business venture presumed that he must have caused the venture to fail on purpose in order to harm her family in some way. She has never got on well with her brother who is 9 years older and who Jeannie describes as always having been 'clever and scary'. She also tries to shout back at the voice, but this does not have the desired effect of making it quiet.

A *formulation* could include the following:

Jeannie has never got on very well with her older distant brother, whom she has always perceived as threatening. She may have grown up with an assumption that: 'others are not to be trusted'. She probably has a predisposition towards psychosis, which appears to have been precipitated by the bullying, an event that may have also reinforced her assumption. The auditory hallucinations that she experienced contained persecutory themes that relate to her distrust of others and, not surprisingly, focus on her brother and reinforce her belief that he is 'evil'. She believes what the voice tells her – it must be right as it knows everything that has gone on in the past and she has no reason to doubt it. She views the voice as very powerful and uncontrollable. Jeannie attempts to silence the voice by shouting at it, but this fails. She begins to misinterpret the mainly neutral actions of others (her brother in particular) as evidence that they would like to intentionally harm her (egocentric and intentionalising bias). She listens in to conversations between her mother and others for evidence that her brother really does have harmful intent, and discounts evidence pointing to the fact that he does not (selective abstraction). Her way of coping with the persecutory beliefs is to avoid her brother and, to a lesser extent, everyone else. This does not provide the scenarios where Jeannie is forced to consider that her brother does not wish to harm her.

The treatment

In CBT for psychosis, it is essential to carefully foster a trusting therapeutic alliance. While this is true for all CBT, it is particularly the case in psychosis due to trust issues and the potential for misinterpretation. Some patients will have had the experience of enforced hospitalisation and other treatments that have resulted in the breakdown of trust with professionals. This must particularly be borne in mind when the therapist is from a profession that may be perceived by the patient as a threat. It has been suggested that CBT works best in this area when there is an explicit 'common purpose' agreed upon between the patient and therapist at the beginning of the therapy such as 'reducing the distress I feel because of my belief' (Chadwick *et al*, 1996).

CBT for *hallucinations* generally includes the following:

- an exploration into the *attributes of the voice(s)*. In particular this needs to concentrate on whether the patient views their voice(s) as all-powerful and with the ability to control and perhaps inflict harm. This needs to be addressed early in therapy, as the patient may be reluctant to deal with an entity that they perceive as so threatening, and so may even fall out of therapy (Chadwick *et al*, 1996)
- by extension, the patient may be encouraged to carefully experiment with *not doing what is demanded* by the voice and then observing whether the catastrophic predictions truly occur or not. In this way the patient can be coached to simply

allow the voice to say what it wants, but to not react to it either emotionally or behaviourally. This type of experimentation can therefore not only lead to behavioural change but also change the beliefs that the patient holds about the voice – how can it be all-powerful if it fails to carry out the threats when its instructions are ignored?

- there needs to be an exploration of the identity of the voice(s). In particular, patients need to be encouraged to see the voices as having their *origins in their thoughts*, despite being perceived by the brain as an external perception

- the above 'normalisation' of hallucinations can be assisted by *psycho-education*. Patients are encouraged to learn more about the ways that hallucinations are experienced and dealt with by others. In the UK a *Hearing Voices* network explores these issues in a group format and allows patients to access information that might not be accepted from a professional. This group approach can also act to *reduce the stigma associated with psychosis* (Romme and Escher, 1994)

- behavioural experiments may identify *helpful modifiers* – situations or behaviours that allow the hallucinations to become either quieter or less distressing for the patient. Some states such as tiredness or hunger are identified as precipitants of the voice(s), and through this understanding, clients can try and regularise their sleeping and eating habits. Some patients learn that gently listening to the voices and not getting emotional and shouting back helps them not to become distressed by them. They therefore develop a helpful *coping repertoire*. Unhelpful coping strategies such as the routine and excessive use of *avoidance* need to be addressed. Isolation, times spent ruminating about the voices, and boredom may have exacerbated the hallucinations. Alternatively, psychotic experiences can result in depression that can itself make either the hallucinations or the emotional reaction to the voices much worse. Where safe, the isolation can be gradually reduced, although not to the point that it results in over-stimulation.

CBT for *delusions* generally includes the following:

- if the aim is to *reduce the intensity of the delusional belief* (or system of belief), then the basic principle is the gathering of evidence to be able to weigh up whether the beliefs are really true. This evidence gathering should, as far as possible, come from the patient. It is important not to argue or directly confront the delusional belief with the patient, as this is likely to make the patient react by becoming more defensive and result in the belief becoming more entrenched (Milton *et al*, 1978)

- generally, *the evidence that supports or refutes the belief system* is assessed before looking face-on at the validity of the delusional belief itself (Kingdon and Turkington, 1998). Therefore, if the delusional belief is that a neighbour is using soap products to poison the patient, then the work may start by looking at the true potential danger of soap products rather than looking at the intent of the neighbour *per se*

- when the delusional beliefs are directly addressed, the more *peripheral beliefs* in the overall system are addressed first. These tend to be associated with less emotion, and elicit less of the same defensive reaction. The central delusions are addressed later when the client is more trusting of the therapist and familiar with the therapy (Kingdon and Turkington, 1998). Therefore, in the example above, the belief that the neighbour tried to 'distress' the patient two years ago using excessive noise may be looked at first, before addressing the issue of the current 'poisoning'.

A key delusion that Jeannie held was that her brother was 'evil'. This was not addressed early in therapy as it was seen as too emotive. Initially, the therapist concentrated on the therapeutic relationship, and in time it was agreed that they would examine the beliefs that her brother had poisoned perfume and had moved tablets in order to tempt her to kill herself. She agreed to compare the smell of her perfume with other bottles of the same brand. She also thought that her mother still had the receipt and decided to ask her to show her it to check that the receipt matched the perfume. After Jeannie predicted that it would burn the skin if worn, her mother (and therapist) kindly agreed to try putting the perfume on their skin first. When the patient's belief about the perfume being dangerous was re-rated, it dropped from 100% down to 20%. Similar experiments and examination of the evidence were applied to other peripheral delusional beliefs, which contributed to her central belief that her brother was evil, and wanted to kill her.

Early on in treatment, the therapist also explained that the voice was an extension of her thoughts and that this was how the voice knew about Jeannie's past rather than any inherent power held by the voice. It took some time for Jeannie to begin to acknowledge this possibility, and this came only after she agreed to join a local *Hearing Voices* support group. Jeannie was able to make the voice worse by talking about distressing things from her past, and then make the voice better again by relaxing, trying not to resist the voice, and reminding herself that they were only 'verbalised thoughts'. This challenged the view that the voice was 'all-powerful', and 'uncontrollable'. Jeannie told the therapist that this experiment had helped her feel much better.

Finally, the accumulation of evidence regarding the identity and characteristics of the voice allowed Jeannie to begin to address her central delusion that her brother was evil and wanted to kill her. Further evidence was gathered from Jeannie's mother, who again came to the session with Jeannie. In time it was felt by all concerned that it would be safe to arrange fact-finding sessions between the family members including with the brother. *All the involved professionals only did this after a careful risk assessment.* In these sessions peripheral supporting information was challenged, and this helped to reduce the conviction of the delusional beliefs that Jeannie held about her brother. This occurred despite the fact that her voices still intermittently told her that he was 'evil'. She continued to attend the *Hearing Voices* group and at most times was able to ignore the voices.

MAIN POINTS

- Hallucinatory experiences are more common in the general population than previously thought. Furthermore, delusions are more often 'understandable' to some degree than previously acknowledged.
- Cognitive errors such as making personal and external attributions for negative events play a part in the maintenance of delusions and hallucinations.
- Although there may be a biological predisposition to hearing voices, the patient's responses to them probably play a part in their maintenance. Both distraction and actively talking back at the voices tend to exacerbate them.
- Encouraging patients to accept the voices, not to be overly emotional about them and not to distract themselves often helps the patient to cope better with them.
- Treatment often incorporates behavioural experiments to test out some of the beliefs the patient holds about the voice(s). These include testing out whether the voice(s) are as powerful as they say, and testing out which environmental factors make them better and worse.
- Work with psychotic patients – in particular work that challenges delusional systems – requires a trusting therapeutic relationship. Before the central delusional beliefs are challenged, the therapy concentrates both on challenging the supporting evidence for the central delusions, and on challenging any other peripheral delusional beliefs.

Further reading

- Chadwick P and Birchwood M (1994) The omnipotence of voices. A cognitive approach to auditory hallucinations. *British Journal of Psychiatry* **164**: 190–201.
- Chadwick P, Birchwood M and Trower P (1996) *Cognitive Therapy for Delusions, Voices and Paranoia*. Chichester: Wiley.
- Kingdon D and Turkington D (1998) Cognitive behaviour therapy of schizophrenia. In: Wykes T, Tarrier N and Lewis S (eds) *Outcome and Innovation in Psychological Treatment of Schizophrenia*. Chichester: Wiley, pp. 59–79.

Chapter 15

Cognitive behavioural therapy applied to borderline personality disorder

---

The models • Assessment and formulation • The treatment

The models

Three major cognitive behavioural approaches to borderline personality disorder (BPD) are taken by Aaron T. Beck (*see* Beck *et al*, 1990, 2004), Jeff Young (schema therapy, *see* Young *et al*, 2003) and Marsha Linehan (dialectical behaviour therapy (DBT), *see* Linehan, 1993). This chapter will attempt to present only a very basic overview of these three approaches. Those requiring further information need to access the references provided in the further reading section at the end of this chapter. A key concept inherent in all three approaches is that of the 'schema'. Schemas have been defined as: 'organized elements of past reactions and experience that form a relatively cohesive and persistent body of knowledge capable of guiding subsequent perception and appraisals' (Segal, 1988, p. 147). Put simply, schemas can be seen as the lens through which we interpret the world, where that lens has been shaped by past experiences.

Pretzer and Beck (2004) outline the effects of an abusive early environment on schemas and subsequent behaviours. Not surprisingly, clients with BPD usually view the *world as 'dangerous' and other people as 'untrustworthy'*. They respond by being hyper-vigilant to threats, and because of this frequently interpret the neutral actions of others as threatening, resulting in paranoia and aggression. They also *view themselves as weak or vulnerable*, and because of this may form dependent relationships with others. The dependency frequently makes the *relationships unstable*, exacerbated by the BPD patient's distrust of others and *poor ability to tolerate frustration*. They frequently also use *avoidance* as a predominant strategy. This avoidance extends not only to places or people, but also to the strong emotions that people with BPD experience. The avoidance of people and places reinforces the client's view that the situation must be threatening. The fear and avoidance of strong emotions place those with BPD at risk of a variety of behaviours such as *alcohol and drug abuse* and other *dangerous activities* undertaken to mask these emotions. Unfortunately, the emotions 'then suddenly manifest themselves at full intensity' (Pretzer and Beck, 2004, p. 310). This reinforces the BPD client's view that their *emotions are unacceptable and dangerous*, and they step up their avoidance strategies. Other factors influence the BPD presentation, including *poor problem-solving skills* and a tendency to engage in *dichotomous thinking* (all or nothing thinking). The latter intensifies the emotions experienced and further negatively influences the quality of relationships.

Young's model of treatment is not in conflict with any of the above (Young *et al*, 2003). However, the emphasis in schema-focused therapy is on *'early maladaptive schemas'* (EMS). Young marks these out as different from most people's schemas, in that they tend to be formed in response to early abusive or neglectful situations, they are generally maladaptive to the client's adult surroundings and they are highly resistant to change. They may have been adaptive, and indeed essential, to the childhood environment, but their perseverance and rigidity in the adult context is disabling for the individual. Young links groups (called *'domains'*) of EMS to corresponding aversive life circumstances. He surmises that we all have a number of schemas, but at any time some will be active and others dormant. So, if we have a schema with a theme of 'failure' this may be dormant for much of the time but activated by characteristic *triggers* such as exam time. When certain schemas are activated, we have characteristic associated styles of thinking, feeling and behaving. Young calls these characteristic patterns of responding: *'schema modes'*. Finally, Young uses the term *'schema processes'* to describe the ways in which we all act to maintain our preformed schemas, thus making them resistant to change. Interpreting events in a way that is in keeping with our schema is one way in which our schemas are not challenged – 'I didn't want to pass the exams that much anyway'. Another process is to simply avoid the situations and thoughts that could challenge them – such as deciding not to work for an exam.

The DBT model is based on elements from behavioural therapy, Zen Buddhism, and dialectical philosophy. A *dialectical viewpoint* refers to the ability to see a situation from polar opposite perspectives at any given time. Linehan noted that BPD clients have difficulty taking *opposite (dialectical) perspectives*, and they are prone to *dichotomous* 'all or nothing' thinking. The result of this is that attitudes and affect change suddenly. The child fails to learn control of its own emotions resulting in *'emotional dysregulation'*, and there is a tendency for this to cause marked distortions and errors in thinking. BPD is described as originating in *'invalidating environments'* in childhood (in addition to a contributory biological origin). Linehan (1993) describes how, through neglect, some clients with BPD have not been taught to *label emotions* or to *problem solve*. Furthermore, attempts to elicit child–parent interactions may have been met with a lack of interest, so that only a significant escalation of behaviours led to these attention needs being met. The adult presentation of the BPD may therefore be in part due to *unhelpful learned behaviours*.

Assessment and formulation

The following information will be sought regarding BPD:

- the main *presenting features* of BPD described in ICD-10 or DSM-IV should be enquired into, including evidence of periods of dissociation and associated self-harming behaviours, and a tendency to engage in very intense but insecure relationships
- as always, what are the ways in which BPD has *affected the patient's life*? The interaction between BPD and environment will be two-way and complex

- is there any *dependency on alcohol or illicit drugs* and *other mental health conditions* such as depression?
- does the patient have *poor problem-solving skills* and evidence of unhelpful behaviour responses, such as a tendency to respond using aggression?
- what are the *maintaining factors* for these behaviours? For example, is the patient respected for their ability to threaten aggression?
- what are the likely *dysfunctional assumptions* and *schemas*? This is sometimes clear at interview, but may need to be surmised based on the patient's behaviour in current and past situations
- is there evidence of *clear dichotomous thinking*, including within the interview situation?
- is there evidence of childhood '*invalidating environments*' or *abuse*?
- is there evidence of re-experiencing symptoms such as complex 'flashbacks' from early traumas such as abuse, and other features of 'complex PTSD'?

Example

Deborah is a 23-year-old woman with a diagnosis of BPD, which she was given in adult services after 5 years' care in the child and adolescent mental health services (where she had a diagnosis of 'conduct disorder'). She had cut herself and taken overdoses since the age of 14. She had a history of severe emotional, physical and sexual abuse in a chaotic family environment. Deborah hated herself and had a rule that she 'never trusted anyone'. She required short inpatient stays in hospital during times of crisis. These periods could be predicted to some extent – they were generally times of conflict with her partner who also had a diagnosis of BPD, and during periods when she was reminded of the sexual abuse in her early childhood at the hands of her stepfather. October, the time of her stepfather's death, was a period when Deborah invariably required a period of inpatient stay. Deborah was not popular on the ward as she invariably got into arguments with other patients, and at times these had become violent. She also used a variety of illicit drugs and misused alcohol. When she was drunk she invariably became hostile and was prone to severe bouts of self-harm. During periods of severe crisis she would appear distant and pale, and would sit rocking for long periods. However, Deborah denied having had any re-experiencing symptoms such as flashbacks relating to the abuse in her childhood. Deborah's home was bare with sparse furniture. During crisis periods at home, Deborah's partner informed staff that she would sit alone in a cold dark room deliberating over her decision whether to kill herself or not. He regretted that the couple had 'little quality of life'.

A *formulation* would include the following:

Deborah has clear features of BPD, including periods of intense affect and dissociation that the patient attempts to mask using a variety of behaviours. These have included self-harming behaviours, alcohol and multiple illicit drug misuse, and the use of aggression towards herself. When gripped by a period of intense emotion and dissociation, Deborah does not use strategies of self-care that nurture or that successfully curtail her affect. The behavioural strategies that she does use, such as drug use, temporarily allow her to avoid her negative affect, but result in further problems such as drug dependency needs with which Deborah is poorly equipped to cope. She grew up in an invalidating environment that probably failed to teach Deborah to label and identify her own emotions, to problem solve and to use self-care techniques. She was taught verbal and physical aggression as a predominant coping strategy. While this may have been necessary in her childhood environment, it results in hostile and insecure relationships. Deborah holds a dysfunctional assumption that if she 'trusts others they will let her down'. She has schemas regarding others as 'threatening' and herself as 'vulnerable' and 'worthless'. Her dysfunctional assumptions and schemas result in Deborah misinterpreting the behaviours of others, including her partner and hospital staff, as hostile, and she responds in a predictably hostile manner. Her hostility has resulted in the breakdown of a variety of relationships. These broken relationships have in turn reinforced Deborah's view that she must be worthless, that others are not to be trusted, and that she is vulnerable. There is no evidence of concurrent illnesses, although there is a history of depression, no doubt contributed to by the poor problem-solving and self-care skills and the associated negative life events.

The treatment

There are a number of general differences between the general CBT approach to BPD and the approach taken towards Axis 1 disorders (Davidson, 2000). For example, in BPD the client is usually seen for a longer period – normally for at least 9 months. Therapy is slower due to the entrenched nature of many of the beliefs and behaviours, and the relationship between the client and therapist forms a more important part of the therapy. There is also more of an emphasis on past events and relationships in the context of understanding current problems than is the case for the 'here and now' traditional CBT approach for Axis 1 disorders. The specific approach taken differs depending on which of the three aforementioned models are used.

The 'Beckian' CBT approach for BPD

There is significant overlap between the techniques used in CBT for depression and anxiety and those used for BPD. As before, the therapy needs to be based upon a formulation that has been jointly agreed between the client and the therapist. Similarly, DTRs are used to help the client challenge some of the unhelpful automatic thoughts that drive unhelpful behaviours. There is an emphasis on addressing and correcting the dichotomous 'all or nothing' thinking style so commonly used by BPD clients. A *detailed analysis of some of the unhelpful behaviours* is made, and the client and therapist set up experiments to see if the1 ways of dealing with these situations. In particular, *underdeveloped beh* as self-nurturing behaviours during periods of distress are discussed a (Davidson, 2000). These are then repeatedly practised so that they are integrateu into the client's repertoire of behaviours for the future. Unhelpful overdeveloped behaviours, such as the use of aggression, are identified. Experimentation with reducing their use can then be attempted (Davidson, 2000). There is also an emphasis on testing out some of the *underlying dysfunctional assumptions* and *schemas* held by the client. Where an underlying schema is particularly influential (e.g. belief in one's self as defective) then challenging this will form the greater part of the content of therapy. One way of doing this is by gathering data that contradict this belief and, importantly, to then create a new more positive and realistic belief. Data that confirm this new belief can then be collected over time using a 'positive belief log' (Beck *et al*, 1990; Padesky, 1994). For example, if a new agreed belief is: 'I'm considerate', then the client can jot down incidents, behaviours and events daily in this log that give evidence of this belief – perhaps helping a neighbour with a problem or spending time on the phone with a distressed relative.

The schema therapy approach for BPD

There is an *'assessment' phase* and a *'change' phase*. The identification of the most relevant negative schemas for the client is the main focus of the assessment phase, while attempting to change them is the primary focus of the change phase. This is similar to the traditional cognitive behavioural approach to BPD, although schema therapy uses different techniques to achieve schema change. Young describes schema therapy as 'integrated', in that it uses methods from other non-cognitive behavioural models of therapy such as gestalt and object relations (Young *et al*, 2003). The therapist not only identifies the schemas but also attempts to activate them (*schema activation*), by asking the client to imagine scenes (normally from childhood) associated with the schema in question. For example, one client with a defectiveness/shame schema imagined and described to the therapist a particularly distressing period when his father had bullied him. The recalled image may be 'altered' by the client and the therapist working together by imagining the events turning out differently in some way. This client might imagine himself standing up to his father, or imagine the therapist intervening in the scene, standing up to his father for him.

The DBT approach for BPD

In common with the underlying model, DBT treatments use elements drawn from behavioural therapy, Zen Buddhism, and dialectical philosophy. In terms of *behavioural therapy*, the client and therapist carry out detailed behavioural analyses of the steps leading up to the acting out of key behaviours. For example, an episode of self-harm may be examined in detail. The sequence of thoughts, behaviours and emotions that led up to the self-harm will be drawn out and analysed. The client will be asked if the situation could have been viewed and dealt with differently. *Zen techniques* used include *'mindfulness'*. This is a meditational technique whereby the person focuses on the current 'moment' and the environment around them, as opposed to focusing on their internal thoughts and emotions. Finally, the therapist aims to teach (and model) the capacity to hold opposite viewpoints on a subject at the same time (*dialectic approach*). A comprehensive DBT treatment comprises both individual *one-to-one* psychotherapy sessions and attendance at *groups* that aim to teach skills. It is part of the treatment model that there should be 24-hour emergency access to the therapist (supported by a consultation team of other therapists). This is to help with the coaching of new skills during periods of crises – *'in vivo coaching'*. However, this service is both financially and therapist intensive, and in the UK is rarely incorporated fully into mental health services, which tend to use only some elements of the DBT approach such as DBT-based groups.

Deborah agreed to enter into a trial of CBT for BPD that was based upon 'Beckian' principles. The first sessions were difficult, and Deborah left two of them mid-session screaming that the therapist was 'not going to be of any help'. Despite this, the therapist never felt physically under threat and Deborah always came back for more sessions. Deborah was allowed to take her time to 'tell her story', and collaboratively a formulation was drawn out outlining Deborah's schemas and some of her dysfunctional assumptions. Her predominant coping behaviours were also listed in terms of those that were 'overdeveloped', such as her ability to 'stand up for her rights' using aggression, and those that were underdeveloped, such as self-nurturing behaviours. She understood her coping strategies as ways of coping with highly distressing emotions, but agreed that other coping strategies may serve her better. Deborah tried different ways of trying to self-soothe that did not involve aggression, drugs or alcohol, or severe self-harm. She tried a number of techniques including creating a soothing environment at home, having reassuring videos available if needed, and phoning a local crisis hotline for 'a chat'. A regular crisis admission was arranged for the second week in October. Many sessions were also spent assessing the evidence both for and against her belief (schema) that she was 'worthless' and 'vulnerable'. Deborah kept a file that outlined all the evidence. Evidence was written down about events that occurred between sessions and from the results of specific tasks. One such task was to ask a number of trusted friends how they assessed a person's worth, and then deliberating upon the results. The therapy lasted for 18 months and although there was no 'cure' at the end, the frequency of Deborah's admissions to hospital and episodes of overdosing had fallen by two-thirds in the final 6 months of therapy, and was maintained at this lower level in the 6 months after therapy had ended.

MAIN POINTS
- Three major forms of therapy for BPD based upon cognitive and behavioural principles are DBT (Linehan), 'Beckian CBT' and Schema Therapy (Young).
- Patients with BPD often hold schemas that have been shaped by early abusive, neglectful, or 'invalidating' environments. These schemas are

often that the world is a threat, that others cannot be trusted and that they themselves are 'worthless'.

- The presenting problems are often connected with a poor ability to tolerate distress, and emotional instability.
- Unhelpful coping strategies such as substance misuse, aggression, self-harm and avoidance are themselves connected with the schemas and emotional dyscontrol.
- Schema therapy focuses on 'early-maladaptive schemas', 'schema modes' and 'schema processes'.
- The use and manipulation of imagery is a major part of schema therapy.
- DBT uses elements of behaviour therapy, Buddhism and 'dialectical philosophy'.
- DBT encourages the reduction of 'all-or-nothing' thinking. It is administered in individual one-to-one therapy in association with group education formats. 'Mindfulness' is also practised.
- The 'Beckian' model of treatment emphasises schema change in addition to the adoption of new previously underdeveloped coping strategies such as self-care. It also encourages the reduction of overdeveloped unhelpful coping strategies, such as aggression and self-harming.

Further reading

- Beck AT, Freeman A, Davis D *et al.* (2004) *Cognitive Therapy of Personality Disorders* (2e). New York: Guilford Press.
- Davidson K (2000) *Cognitive Therapy for Personality Disorders: a guide for therapists.* Oxford: Butterworth-Heinemann.
- Linehan MM (1993) *Cognitive-behavioural Treatment of Borderline Personality Disorder.* New York: Guilford Press.
- Young JE, Klosko JS and Weishaar ME (2003) *Schema Therapy: a practitioner's guide.* New York: Guilford Press.

References

Acierno R, Hersen M, Van Hasselt VB *et al.* (1994) Review of the validation and dissemination of eye-movement desensitization and reprocessing: A scientific and ethical dilemma. *Clinical Psychology Review* 14: 287–99.

Agras WS, Walsh T, Fairburn CG, Wilson GT and Kraemer HC (2000) A multicentre comparison of cognitive-behavioural therapy and interpersonal psychotherapy for bulimia nervosa. *Archives of General Psychiatry* 57: 459–66.

American Psychiatric Association (2000) Practice guideline for the treatment of patients with major depressive disorder (revision). *American Journal of Psychiatry* 157 (suppl. 4): 1–45.

American Psychiatric Association (2001) Practice guideline for the treatment of patients with borderline personality disorder. *American Journal of Psychiatry* 158(suppl): 1–52.

American Psychiatric Association (1994) *Diagnostic and Statistical Manual of Mental Disorders* (4e). Washington DC: American Psychiatric Association.

Antony MM and Barlow DH (2002) Specific phobias. In: Barlow DH (ed) *Anxiety and its Disorders: the nature and treatment of anxiety and panic* (2e). New York: Guilford Press, pp. 380–417.

Ashworth P, Williams C and Blackburn I-M (1999) What becomes of cognitive therapy trainees? A survey of trainees' opinions and current clinical practice after postgraduate cognitive therapy training. *Behavioural and Cognitive Psychotherapy* 27: 267–77.

Ayllon T and Azrin N (1968) *The Token Economy*. New York: Appleton Century Crofts.

Bach P and Hayes S (2002) The use of acceptance and commitment therapy to prevent the rehospitalization of psychotic patients: a randomized controlled trial. *Journal of Consulting and Clinical Psychology* 70: 1129–39.

Bandura A (1977a) *Social Learning Theory*. Englewood Cliffs, NJ: Prentice-Hall.

Bandura A (1977b) Self-efficacy: towards a unifying theory of behavioural change. *Psychological Review* 84: 191–215.

Barkham M, Evans C, Margison F *et al.* (1998) The rationale for developing and implementing core outcome batteries for routine use in service settings and psychotherapy outcome research. *Journal of Mental Health* 7: 21–35.

Barlow DH, Gorman JM, Shear MK and Woods SW (2000) Cognitive-behavioural therapy, imipramine, or their combination for panic disorder: A randomized controlled trial. *Journal of the American Medical Association* 283: 2529–36.

Barrowclough C, Tarrier N, Lewis S *et al.* (1999) Randomised controlled effectiveness trial of a needs-based psychosocial intervention service for carers of people with schizophrenia. *British Journal of Psychiatry*, 174: 505–11.

Basco MR and Rush AJ (1996) *Cognitive-behavioural Therapy for Bipolar Disorder*. New York: Guilford.

Bateman A and Fonagy P (1999) The effectiveness of partial hospitalization in the treatment of borderline personality disorder – a randomized controlled trial. *American Journal of Psychiatry* 156: 1563–9.

Bateman A and Fonagy P (2001) Treatment of borderline personality disorder with psychoanalytically orientated partial hospitalization: an 18-month follow-up. *American Journal of Psychiatry* 158: 36–42.

Bateman A and Fonagy P (2003) Health service utilization costs for borderline personality disorder patients treated with psychoanalytically orientated partial hospitalization versus general psychiatric care. *American Journal of Psychiatry*, 160: 169–71.

Beck AT (1967) *Depression: Clinical, Experimental and Theoretical Aspects.* New York: Harper Row.

Beck AT (1976) *Cognitive Therapy and the Emotional Disorders.* New York: International Universities Press.

Beck AT (1988) *Love is Never Enough.* New York: Harper Row.

Beck AT and Clark DA (1988) Anxiety and depression: an information processing perspective. *Anxiety Research* 1: 23–36.

Beck AT, Emery G and Greenberg RL (1985) *Anxiety Disorders and Phobias: a cognitive perspective.* New York: Basic Books.

Beck AT, Epstein N, Brown *et al.* (1988) An inventory for measuring clinical anxiety: psychometric properties. *Journal of Consulting and Clinical Psychology* 56: 893–7.

Beck AT and Freeman A and Associates (1990) *Cognitive Therapy of Personality Disorders.* New York: Guilford Press.

Beck AT, Freeman A, Davis D *et al.* (2004) *Cognitive Therapy of Personality Disorders* (2e). New York: Guilford Press.

Beck AT, Rush AJ, Shaw BF and Emery G (1979) *Cognitive Therapy of Depression.* New York: Guilford Press.

Beck AT, Steer RA, Brown GK (1996) *Beck Depression Inventory-II: Manual.* San Antonio: The Psychological Corporation.

Beck AT, Weissman A, Lester D *et al.* (1974) The measurement of pessimism: The Hopelessness Scale. *Journal of Consulting and Clinical Psychology* 42: 861–5.

Bennett-Levy J, Butler G, Fennel M *et al.* (eds) (2004) *Oxford Guide to Behavioural Experiments in Cognitive Therapy.* Oxford: Oxford University Press.

Birchwood M and Trower P (2006) The future of cognitive-behavioural therapy for psychosis: not a quasi-neuroleptic. *British Journal of Psychiatry* 188: 107–8.

Blackburn I-M and Twaddle V (1996) *Cognitive Therapy in Action: a practitioner's casebook.* London: Souvenir Press.

Borkovec TD (1994) The nature, functions, and origins of worry. In: Davey GCL and Tallis F (eds) *Worrying: perspectives on theory, assessment, and treatment.* New York: Springer Publishing Company, pp. 117–27.

Borkovec TD and Ruscio AM (2001) Psychotherapy for generalized anxiety disorder. *Journal of Clinical Psychiatry* 62(suppl 11): 37–42; discussion: 43–5.

Bower P and Gilbody S (2005) Stepped care in psychological therapies: access, effectiveness and efficiency. Narrative literature review. *British Journal of Psychiatry* 186: 11–17.

Bowers W (1990) Treatment of depressed in-patients: cognitive therapy plus medication, relaxation plus medication and medication alone. *British Journal of Psychiatry* 156: 73–8.

Bradley R, Greene J, Russ E, Dutra L and Westen D (2005) A multidimensional meta-analysis of psychotherapy for PTSD. *American Journal of Psychiatry* 162: 214–27.

Braga DT, Cordioli AV, Niederauer K and Manfro GG (2005) Cognitive-behavioral group therapy for obsessive-compulsive disorder: a 1-year follow-up. *Acta Psychiatrica Scandinavica* 112: 180–6.

Brown D and Pedder J (1979) *Introduction to Psychotherapy.* London: Tavistock Publications.

Burns D and Auerbach A (1996) Therapeutic empathy in cognitive-behavioral therapy: Does it really make a difference? In P Salkovskis (ed) *Frontiers of Cognitive Therapy.* New York: Guilford Press, pp. 135–64.

Carter JC and Fairburn CG (1998) Cognitive-behavioural self-help for binge eating disorder: a controlled effectiveness study. *Journal of Consulting and Clinical Psychology* 66: 616–23.

Chadwick P and Birchwood M (1994) The omnipotence of voices. A cognitive approach to auditory hallucinations. *British Journal of Psychiatry* 164: 190–201.

Chadwick P, Birchwood M and Trower P (1996) *Cognitive Therapy for Delusions, Voices and Paranoia.* Chichester: Wiley.

Chambless DL and Gillis MM (1993) Cognitive therapy of anxiety disorders. *Journal of Consulting and Clinical Psychology* **61**: 248–60.

Chambless DL and Peterman M (2004) Evidence on cognitive-behavioral therapy for generalized anxiety disorder and panic disorder: The second decade. In: RL Leahy (ed.) *Contemporary Cognitive Therapy*. New York: Guilford, pp. 86–115.

Churchill R, Hunot V, Corney R *et al.* (2001) A systematic review of controlled trials of the effectiveness and the cost-effectiveness of brief psychological treatments for depression. *Health Technology Assessment* **5**: 1–173.

Clark DM (1986a) A cognitive approach to panic. *Behaviour Research and Therapy* **24**: 461–70.

Clark DM (1986b) Cognitive therapy for anxiety. *Behavioural Psychotherapy* **14**: 283–94.

Clark DM (1989) Anxiety states: panic and generalised anxiety. In: Hawton K, PM, Salkovskis PM, Kirk J and Clark DM (eds) *Cognitive Behaviour Therapy*. Oxford: Oxford University Press, pp. 52–96.

Clark DA (2004) Cognitive-behavioral theory and treatment of obsessive-compulsive disorder: past contributions and current developments. In: Leahy R (ed) *Contemporary Cognitive Therapy*. New York: Guilford, pp. 161–83.

Clark DM and Ehlers A (2004) Posttraumatic Stress Disorder: From cognitive theory to therapy. In: Leahy R (ed) *Contemporary Cognitive Therapy*. New York: Guilford, pp. 141–160.

Clark DM, Salkovskis PM, Hackmann A *et al.* (1999) Brief cognitive therapy for panic disorder: a randomized controlled trial. *Journal of Consulting and Clinical Psychology* **67**: 583–9.

Clark DM and Teasdale JD (1985) Constraints on the effects of mood on memory. *Journal of Personality and Social Psychology* **48**: 1595–608.

Clarkin JF, Glick ID, Haas GL *et al.* (1990) A randomized clinical trial of inpatient family interventions: V. Results for affective disorders. *Journal of Affective Disorders* **18**: 17–28.

Collins English Dictionary: essential edition. (2003) Glasgow: Harper Collins Publishers.

Cottraux J, Note I, Albuisson E *et al.* (2000) Cognitive behaviour therapy versus supportive therapy in social phobia: a randomized controlled trial. *Psychotherapy and Psychosomatics* **69**: 137–46.

Cuijpers P (1997) Bibliotherapy in unipolar depression: A meta-analysis. *Journal of Behaviour Therapy and Experimental Psychiatry* **28**: 139–47.

Dare C, Eisler I, Russell G, Treasure J and Dodge L (2001) Psychological therapies for adults with anorexia nervosa: randomised controlled trial of out-patient treatments. *British Journal of Psychiatry* **178**: 216–21.

Davidson K (2000) *Cognitive Therapy for Personality Disorders: a guide for therapists*. Oxford: Butterworth-Heinemann.

Davidson K, Tyrer P, Gumley A *et al.* (2006a) A randomized controlled trial of cognitive behaviour therapy for borderline personality disorder: rationale for trial, method and description of sample. *Journal of Personality Disorders* **20**: 431–49.

Davidson K, Norrie J, Tyrer P *et al.* (2006b) The effectiveness of cognitive behaviour therapy for borderline personality disorder: results from the BOSCOT trial . *Journal of Personality Disorders* **20**: 450–65.

DeRubeis RJ, Gelfand LA, Tang, TZ *et al.* (1999) Medications versus cognitive behavioral therapy for severely depressed outpatients: Mega-analysis of four randomized comparisons. *American Journal of Psychiatry* **156**: 1007–13.

DeRubeis RJ, Hollon, SD, Amsterdam JD *et al.* (2005) Cognitive therapy vs medications in the treatment of moderate to severe depression. *Archives of General Psychiatry* **62**: 409–16.

Drury V, Birchwood M and Cochrane R (2000) Cognitive therapy and recovery from acute psychosis: a controlled trial: III. Five-year follow-up. *British Journal of Psychiatry* **177**: 8–14.

Drury V, Birchwood M, Cochrane R and Macmillan F (1996a) Cognitive therapy and recovery from acute psychosis: a controlled trial: I. impact on psychotic symptoms. *British Journal of Psychiatry* **169**: 593–601.

Drury V, Birchwood M, Cochrane R and Macmillan F (1996b) Cognitive therapy and recovery from acute psychosis: a controlled trial: II. impact on recovery time. *British Journal of Psychiatry* **169**: 602–607.

Durham RC, Murphy T, Allan T *et al.* (1994) Cognitive therapy, analytic psychotherapy, and anxiety management training for generalized anxiety disorder. *British Journal of Psychiatry* **165**: 315–23.

D'Zurilla TJ (1986) *Problem-solving Therapy: a social competence approach to clinical intervention.* New York: Springer.

Ehlers A and Breuer P (1992) Increased cardiac awareness in panic disorder. *Journal of Abnormal Psychology* **100**: 144–50.

Ehlers A and Clark DM (2000) A cognitive model of persistent posttraumatic stress disorder. *Behaviour Research and Therapy* **38**: 319–45.

Elkin I (1994) The NIMH Treatment of Depression Collaborative Research Program: where we began and where we are. In: Bergin AE and Garfield SL (eds) *Handbook of Psychotherapy and Behaviour Change* (4e). New York: Wiley, pp. 114–42.

Ellis A (1962) *Reason and Emotion in Psychotherapy.* New York: Lyle Stuart.

Emanuels-Zuurveen L and Emmelkamp PM (1996) Individual behavioural-cognitive therapy v. marital therapy for depression in maritally distressed couples. *British Journal of Psychiatry* **169**: 181–8.

Evans MD, Hollon SD, DeRubeis RJ *et al.* (1992) Differential relapse following cognitive therapy and pharmacotherapy for depression. *Archives of General Psychiatry* **49**: 802–8.

Fairburn CG (1997) Eating disorders. In: Clark DM and Fairburn CG (eds) *The Science and Practice of Cognitive Behaviour Therapy.* Oxford: Oxford University Press, pp. 209–41.

Fairburn CG, Jones R, Peveler R *et al.* (1991) Three psychological treatments for bulimia nervosa: a comparative trial. *Archives of General Psychiatry* **48**: 463–9.

Fairburn CG, Norman PA, Welch SL *et al.* (1995) A prospective study of outcome in bulimia nervosa and the long-term effects of three psychological treatments. *Archives of General Psychiatry* **52**: 304–12.

Fairburn CG Shafran R and Cooper Z (1999) A cognitive-behavioural theory of anorexia nervosa. *Behaviour Research and Therapy* **37**: 1–13.

Fedoroff IC and Taylor S (2001) Psychological and pharmacological treatments of social phobia: a meta-analysis. *Journal of Clinical Psychopharmacology* **21**: 311–24.

Fisher PL and Durham RC (1999) Recovery rates in generalized anxiety disorder following psychological therapy: An analysis of clinically significant change in the STAI-T across outcome studies since 1990. *Psychological Medicine* **29**: 1425–34.

Foa EB and Goldstein A (1978) Continuous exposure and complete response prevention in the treatment of obsessive-compulsive neurosis. *Behavior Therapy* **9**: 821–9.

Foa EB, Keane TM and Friedman MJ (eds) (2000) *Effective Treatments for PTSD: practice guidelines from the International Society for Traumatic Stress Studies.* New York: Guilford Press.

Foa EB and Kozak MJ (1986) Emotional processing: theory, research, and clinical implications for anxiety disorders. In: Safran JD and Greenberg LS (eds) *Emotion, Psychotherapy, and Change.* New York: Guilford Press, pp. 21–49.

Foa EB and Kozac MJ (1996) Obsessive-compulsive disorder: long-term outcome of psychological treatment. In: Mavissakalian MR and Prien RF (eds) *Long-term Treatments of Anxiety Disorders.* Washington, DC: American Psychiatric Press, pp. 285–309.

Foa EB, Liebowitz MR, Kozak MJ *et al.* (2005) Randomized, placebo-controlled trial of exposure and ritual prevention, clomipramine, and their combination in the treatment of obsessive-compulsive disorder. *American Journal of Psychiatry* **162**: 151–161.

Foa EB, Rothbaum BO and Furr JM (2003) Augmenting exposure therapy with other CBT procedures. *Psychiatric Annals* **33**: 47–53.

Foa EB, Steketee G and Milby JB (1980) Differential effects of exposure and response prevention in obsessive-compulsive washers. *Journal of Consulting and Clinical Psychology* **48**: 71–9.

Frank E, Kupfer DJ, Thase ME *et al.* (2005) Two-year outcomes for interpersonal and social rhythm therapy in individuals with bipolar I disorder. *Archives of General Psychiatry* **62**: 996–1004.

Frank E, Swartz HA, Mallinger AG *et al.* (1999) Adjunctive psychotherapy for bipolar disorder: Effects of changing treatment modality. *Journal of Abnormal Psychology* **108**: 579–87.

Frank E, Kupfer DJ, Thase ME *et al.* (2005) Two-year outcomes for interpersonal and social rhythm therapy in individuals with bipolar I disorder. *Archives of General Psychiatry* **62**: 996–1004.

Frank J (1971) Therapeutic factors in psychotherapy. *American Journal of Psychotherapy* **25**: 350–61.

Frank JD (1973) *Persuasion and Healing.* Revised edn. Baltimore: John Hopkins Press.

Freeston MH, Ladouceur R, Gagnon F (1997) Cognitive-behavioral treatment of obsessive thoughts: A controlled study. *Journal of Consulting and Clinical Psychology* **65**: 405–413.

Furukawa TA, Wanabe N, Churchill R (2006) Therapy plus antidepressant for panic disorder with or without agoraphobia: Systematic review. *The British Journal of Psychiatry* **188**: 305–12.

Garety PA and Hemsley DR (1994) *Delusions: investigations into the psychology of delusional reasoning.* Oxford: Oxford University Press.

Garner DM (1997) Psychoeducational principles in treatment. In: Garner DM and Garfinkel PE (eds) *Handbook of Treatment for Eating Disorders* (2e). New York: Guilford Press, pp. 145–77.

Garner DM, Vitousek KM and Pike KM (1997) Cognitive-behavior therapy for anorexia nervosa. In: Garner DM and Garfinkel PE (eds) *Handbook of Treatment for Eating Disorders* (2e). New York: Guilford Press, pp. 94–144.

Giesen-Bloo J, van Dyck R, Spinhoven P *et al.* (2006) Outpatient psychotherapy for borderline personality disorder: randomized trial of schema-focused therapy vs. transference-focused psychotherapy. *Archives of General Psychiatry* **63**: 649–58.

Gillespie K, Duffy M, Hackmann A *et al.* (2002) Community based cognitive therapy in the treatment of posttraumatic stress disorder following the Omagh bomb. *Behaviour Research and Therapy* **40**: 345–57.

Goodwin F and Jamison K (1990) *Manic-depressive illness.* Oxford: Oxford University Press.

Gould R, Buckminster S, Pollack M, Otto M and Yap L (1997) Cognitive-behavioural and pharmacological treatment for social phobia: a meta-analysis. *Psychology: Science and Practice* **4**: 291–306.

Greenberger D and Padesky C (1995) *Mind Over Mood: change how you feel by changing the way you think.* London: The Guilford Press.

Gumley A, O'Grady M, McNay L *et al.* (2003) Early intervention for relapse in schizophrenia: results of a 12-month randomized controlled trial of cognitive behavioural therapy. *Psychological Medicine* **33**: 419–31.

Halmi KA, Agras WS, Crow S *et al.* (2005) Predictors of treatment acceptance and completion in anorexia nervosa: Implications for future study design, *Archives of General Psychiatry* **62**: 776–81.

Healy D and Williams JMG (1989) Moods, misattributions and mania: An interaction of biological and psychological factors in the pathogenesis of mania. *Psychiatric Developments* **7**: 49–70.

Heimberg R, Dodge C, Hope D, Kennedy C *et al.* (1990) Cognitive behavioural group treatment for social phobia: comparison with a credible placebo control. *Cognitive Therapy and Research* **14**: 1–23.

Heyman I, Mataix-Cols D and Fineberg NA (2006) Obsessive compulsive disorder: clinical review. *British Medical Journal.* **333**: 424–9.

Hollon SD and DeRubeis RJ (2004) Effectiveness of treatment for depression. In Leahy R (ed) *Contemporary Cognitive Therapy.* New York: Guilford, pp. 45–61.

Hollon SD, DeRubeis RJ, Shelton *et al.* (2005) Prevention of relapse following cognitive therapy vs medications in moderate to severe depression. *Archives of General Psychiatry* **62**: 417–22.

Horowitz MJ (1986) *Stress Response Syndromes* (2e). Northvale, NJ: Jason Aronson.

Horvarth A and Greenberg L (1989) Development and validation of the working alliance inventory. *Journal of Counseling Psychology* **36**: 223–33.

Hughes P (1999) *Dynamic Psychotherapy Explained.* Oxford: Radcliffe Publishing.

Hughes P and Riordan D (2006) *Dynamic Psychotherapy Explained* (2e). Oxford: Radcliffe Publishing.

Janoff-Bulman R (1992) *Shattered Assumptions: towards a new psychology of trauma.* New York: Free Press.

Jones C, Cormac I, Silveira de Mota Neto JI and Campbell C (2004) Cognitive behaviour therapy for schizophrenia (Cochrane Review). *The Cochrane Library, Issue 4.* Oxford: Update Software.

Jorm AF, Korten AE, Jacomb PA *et al.* (1997) Helpfulness of interventions for mental disorders: beliefs of health professionals compared with the general public. *British Journal of Psychiatry* **171**: 233–7.

Kane JM (1996) Treatment resistant schizophrenic patients. *Journal of Clinical Psychiatry* **57**(suppl 9): 35–40.

Keller M, McCullough J, Klein D *et al.* (2000) A comparison of nefazodone, the cognitive behavioural analysis system of psychotherapy, and their combination for the treatment of chronic depression. *New England Journal of Medicine* **342**: 1462–70.

Kenardy JA, Dow MG, Johnston DW *et al.* (2003) A comparison of delivery methods of cognitive-behavioural therapy for panic disorder: an international multicenter trial. *Journal of Consulting and Clinical Psychology* **71**: 1068–75.

Kendall PC and Ingram RE (1987) The future for cognitive assessment of anxiety: let's get specific. In: Michelson L and Ascher LM (eds) *Anxiety and Stress Disorders: cognitive-behavioural assessment and treatment.* New York: Guilford Press, pp. 89–104.

Kinderman P and Bentall RP (1997) Causal attributions in paranoia: Internal, personal and situational attributions for negative events. *Journal of Abnormal Psychology* **106**: 341–5.

Kingdon C (2006) Psychological and social interventions for schizophrenia. *British Medical Journal* **333**: 212–13.

Kingdon D and Turkington D (1994) *Cognitive Behaviour Therapy of Schizophrenia.* New York: Guilford Press.

Kingdon D and Turkington D (1998) Cognitive behaviour therapy of schizophrenia. In: Wykes T, Tarrier N and Lewis S (eds) *Outcome and Innovation in Psychological Treatment of Schizophrenia.* Chichester: Wiley, pp. 59–79.

Kobak KA, Greist JH, Jefferson JW, Katzelnick DJ, Henk HJ, (1998) Behavioural versus pharmacological treatments of obsessive-compulsive disorder: A meta-analysis. *Psycho-pharmacology* **136**: 205–16.

Kolb D (1984) *Experiential learning: experience as source of learning and development.* Englewood Cliffs, NJ: Prentice Hall.

Kuipers E (2000) Psychological treatments for psychosis: evidence based but unavailable. *Psychiatric Rehabilitation Skills* **4**: 249–58.

Lam DH, Jones SH, Hayward P and Bright JA (1999) *Cognitive Therapy for Bipolar Disorder: a therapist's guide to concepts, methods and practice.* Chichester: Wiley.

Lam DH, Hayward P, Watkins E *et al.* (2005a) Outcome of a two-year follow-up of a cognitive therapy of relapse prevention in bipolar disorder. *American Journal of Psychiatry* **162**: 324–9.

Lam DH, McCrone P, Wright K and Kerr N (2005b) Cost-effectiveness of relapse-prevention cognitive therapy for bipolar disorder: 30-month study. *British Journal of Psychiatry* **186**: 500–6.

Lam DH, Watkins ER, Hayward P *et al.* (2003) A randomized controlled study of cognitive therapy for relapse prevention for bipolar affective disorder: outcome of the first year. *Archives of General Psychiatry* **60**: 145–52.

Lam DH and Wong G (1997) Prodromes, coping strategies, insight and social functioning in bipolar affective disorders. *Psychological Medicine* **27**: 1091–100.

Layard, R (2006) *The Case for Psychological Treatment Centres.* Available at http:cep.lse.ac.uk/layard/ (accessed 12 Dec 2006).

Leach C, Lucock, M, Barkham M *et al.* (2005) Assessing risk and emotional disturbance using the CORE-OM and HoNOS outcome measures at the interface between primary and secondary mental healthcare. *Psychiatric Bulletin* **29**: 419–22.

Leahy RL (2003) *Cognitive Therapy Techniques: A practitioner's guide.* New York: Guilford Press.

Leahy RL and Holland SJ (2000) *Treatment Plans and Interventions for Depression and Anxiety Disorders.* New York: Guilford Press.

Leff JP and Vaughn C (1985) *Expressed Emotion in Families.* New York: Guilford Press.

Lewin K (1946) Action research and minority problems. *Journal of Social Issues* **2**: 34–46.

Lewinsohn PM, Munoz RF, Youngren MA and Zeiss AM (1986) Control over depression (2e). Englewood Cliffs, NJ: Prentice Hall.

Lewis S, Tarrier N, Haddock G *et al.* (2002) Randomised controlled trial of cognitive-behavioural therapy in early schizophrenia: acute-phase outcomes. *British Journal of Psychiatry* **43**(suppl): S91–S97.

Lidren DM, Watkins PL, Gould RA *et al.* (1994) A comparison of bibliotherapy and group therapy in the treatment of panic disorder. *Journal of Consulting and Clinical Psychology* **62**: 865–9.

Linehan MM (1993) *Cognitive-behavioural Treatment of Borderline Personality Disorder.* New York: Guilford Press.

Linehan MM, Armstrong HE, Suarez A, Allmon D and Heard H (1991) Cognitive-behaviour treatment of chronically parasuicidal borderline patients. *Archives of General Psychiatry* **48**: 1060–4.

Linehan MM, Comtois KA, Murray AM *et al.* (2006) Two-year randomized controlled trial and follow-up of dialectical behaviour therapy vs. therapy by experts for suicidal behaviours and borderline personality disorder. *Archives of General Psychiatry* **63**: 757–66.

Linehan MM, Heard H and Armstrong HE (1993) Naturalistic follow-up of a behavioural treatment for chronically parasuicidal borderline patients. *Archives of General Psychiatry* **50**: 971–4.

Lovell K, Cox D, Haddock G *et al.* (2006) Telephone administered cognitive behavioural therapy for treatment of obsessive compulsive disorder: randomised controlled non-inferiority trial. *British Medical Journal.* **333**: 883–8.

Lyubomirsky S and Nolen-Hoeksema S (1995) Effects of self-focused rumination on negative thinking and interpersonal problem solving. *Journal of Personality and Social Psychology* **69**: 176–90.

Marks IM, Swinson RP, Basoglu M *et al.* (1993) Alprazolam and exposure alone and combined in panic disorder with agoraphobia. *Journal of Psychiatry* **162**: 776–87.

Mathews A (1997) Information-processing biases in emotional disorders. In: Clark DM and Fairburn CG (eds) *Science and Practice of Cognitive Behaviour Therapy.* Oxford: Oxford University Press, pp. 47–66.

McDermut W, Miller IW and Brown RA (2001) The efficacy of group psychotherapy for depression: A meta-analysis and review of the empirical research. *Clinical Psychology: Science and Practice* **8**: 98–116.

McIntosh V, Jordan J, Carter FA *et al.* (2005) Three psychotherapies for anorexia nervosa: A randomized controlled trial. *American Journal of Psychiatry* **162**: 741–8.

McKenna PJ (2006) Cognitive behaviour therapy is not effective [letter]. *British Medical Journal* **333**: 353.

McLean PD, Whittal ML, Thordarson DS *et al.* (2001) Cognitive versus behaviour therapy in the group treatment of obsessive-compulsive disorder. *Journal of Consulting and Clinical Psychology* **69**: 205–14.

Milton F, Ptwa VK and Hafner RJ (1978) Confrontation vs. belief modification in persistently deluded patients. *British Journal of Psychology* **51**: 127–30.

Moorey S (1996) Cognitive behaviour therapy for whom? *Advances in Psychiatric Treatment* **2**: 17–23.

Moreno P, Méndez X, Sánchez J (2001) Effectiveness of cognitive-behavioural treatment in social phobia: A meta-analytic review. *Psychology in Spain* **5**: 17–25.

Morrison AP (1998) A cognitive analysis of auditory hallucinations: are voices to schizophrenia what bodily sensations are to panic? *Behavioural and Cognitive Psychotherapy* **26**: 289–302.

Morrison AP, French P, Walford L *et al.* (2004) Cognitive therapy for the prevention of psychosis in people at ultra high risk: randomised controlled trial. *British Journal of Psychiatry* **185**: 291–7.

Morrison AP and Haddock G (1997) Self-focused attention in schizophrenic patients and normal subjects: a comparative study. *Personality and Individual Differences* **23**: 937–41.

Mowrer O (1960) *Learning Theory and Behaviour.* New York: Wiley.

Mynors-Wallis LM, Gath DH, Day A and Baker F (2000) Randomised controlled trial of problem solving treatment, antidepressant medication, and combined treatment for major depression in primary care. *British Medical Journal* **320**: 26–30.

National Institute for Health and Clinical Excellence (2002) *Schizophrenia: core interventions in the treatment and management of schizophrenia in primary and secondary care. Clinical Guideline CG001.* London: NICE.

National Institute for Health and Clinical Excellence (2004a) *Depression: management of depression in primary and secondary care. Clinical Guideline CG023.* London: NICE.

National Institute for Health and Clinical Excellence (2004b) *Anxiety: management of anxiety (panic disorder, with or without agoraphobia, and generalised anxiety disorder) in adults in primary, secondary and community care. Clinical Guideline CG022.* London: NICE.

National Institute for Health and Clinical Excellence (2004c) *Eating Disorders: Core interventions in the treatment and management of anorexia nervosa, bulimia nervosa and related eating disorders. Clinical Guideline CG009.* London: NICE.

National Institute for Health and Clinical Excellence (2005a) *Obsessive Compulsive Disorder: Core interventions in the treatment of obsessive compulsive disorder and body dysmorphic disorder. Clinical Guideline CG031.* London: NICE.

National Institute for Health and Clinical Excellence (2005b) *Anxiety: Management of posttraumatic stress disorder in primary, secondary and community care. Clinical Guideline CG026.* London: NICE.

National Institute for Health and Clinical Excellence (2006a) *Computerised cognitive behavioural therapy for depression and anxiety: Guidance. Technology Appraisal TA97.* London: NICE.

National Institute for Health and Clinical Excellence (2006b) *The Management of bipolar disorder in adults, children and adolescents, in primary and secondary care. Clinical Guideline CG038.* London: NICE.Newcastle Cognitive and Behavioural Therapies Centre and the University of Newcastle Upon Tyne (1999) *Manual of the Revised Cognitive Therapy Scale (CTS-R).* Newcastle Upon Tyne, UK.

Nolen-Hoeksema S and Morrow J (1991) A prospective study of depression and posttraumatic stress symptoms after a natural disaster: The 1989 Loma Prieta earthquake. *Journal of Personality and Social Psychology* **61**: 115–21.

Öst LG (1989) One session treatment for specific phobias. *Behaviour Research and Therapy* **27**: 1–7.

Öst, LG, Salkovskis P and Hellstrom K (1991) One session therapist directed exposure vs. self-exposure in the treatment of spider phobia. *Behaviour Therapy* **22** 407–22.

O'Sullivan G and Marks I (1991) Follow-up studies of behavioral treatment of phobic and obsessive compulsive neuroses. *Psychiatric Annals* **21**: 368–73.

Padesky CA (1994) Schema change processes in cognitive therapy. *Clinical Psychology and Psychotherapy* **1**: 267–278.

Paley G and Shapiro DA (2002) Lessons from psychotherapy research for psychological interventions for people with schizophrenia. *British Journal of Medical Psychology* **75**: 5–17.

Palmer B (2004) Bulimia nervosa: 25 years on. *The British Journal of Psychiatry* **185**: 447–8.

Palmer B (2006) Come the revolution. Revisiting: The management of anorexia nervosa. *Advances in Psychiatric Treatment* **12**: 5–12.

Palmer S, Davidson K, Tyrer P *et al.* (2006) The cost-effectiveness of cognitive behaviour therapy for borderline personality disorder: results from the BOSCOT trial. *Journal of Personality Disorders* **20**: 466–81.

Pato MT, Zoka-Kadouch R, Zohar J and Murphy DL (1988) Return of symptoms after desensitization of clomipramine in patients with obsessive-compulsive disorder. *American Journal of Psychiatry* **145**: 1521–5.

Paykel ES (2001) Continuation and maintenance therapy in depression. *British Medical Bulletin* **57**: 145–59.

Paykel ES, Scott J, Teasdale JD *et al.* (1999) Prevention of relapse in residual depression by cognitive therapy: A controlled trial. *Archives of General Psychiatry* **56**: 829–35.

Perry A, Tarrier N, Morriss R, McCarthy E and Limb K (1999) Randomised controlled trial of efficacy of teaching patients with bipolar disorder to identify early symptoms of relapse and obtain treatment. *British Medical Journal* **318**: 139–53.

Persons JB (1989) Cognitive therapy in practice: a case formulation approach. New York: WW Norton and Company.

Pharoah FM, Rathbone J, Mari JJ and Streiner D (2002) Family intervention for schizophrenia (Cochrane Review). *The Cochrane Library, Issue 4.* Oxford: Update Software.

Pike K (1998) Long-term course of anorexia nervosa: Response, relapse, remission, and recovery. *Clinical Psychology Review* **18**: 447–75.

Pike KM, Walsh BT, Vitousek K, Wilson GT and Bauer J (2003) Cognitve behaviour therapy in the post-hospitalisation treatment of anorexia nervosa. *American Journal of Psychiatry* **160**: 2046–9.

Pilling S, Bebbington P, Kuipers E *et al.* (2002) Psychological treatments in schizophrenia: I. Meta-analysis of family intervention and cognitive behaviour therapy. *Psychological Medicine* **32**: 763–82.

Pirraglia PA, Rosen AB, Hermann RC, Olchanski NV and Neumann P (2004) Cost–utility analysis studies of depression management: a systematic review. *American Journal of Psychiatry* **161**: 2155–62.

Polivy J and Herman CP (1995) Dieting and its relation to eating disorders. In K D Brownell & C G Fairburn (eds) *Comprehensive Textbook of Eating Disorders and Obesity.* New York: Guilford Press, pp. 83–86.

Pretzer J and Beck JS (2004) Cognitive therapy of personality disorders: twenty years of progress. In: Leahy RL (ed) *Contemporary Cognitive Therapy.* New York: Guilford Press, pp. 219–318.

Proudfoot J, Goldberg DP, Mann A *et al.* (2003) Computerized, interactive, multimedia cognitive behavioural therapy for anxiety and depression in general practice. *Psychological Medicine* **33**: 217–27.

Rachman S (1980) Emotional processing. *Behaviour Research and Processing* **18**: 51–60.

Rachman S (1997) The evolution of cognitive behaviour therapy. In: Clark DM and Fairburn CG (eds) *Science and Practice of Cognitive Behaviour Therapy*. Oxford: Oxford University Press, pp. 1–26.

Rachman S and Shafran R (1999) Cognitive distortions: thought-action fusion. *Clinical Psychology and Psychotherapy* **6**: 80–5.

Rector NA and Beck AT (2001) Cognitive behavioural therapy for schizophrenia: an empirical review. *Journal of Nervous and Mental Disease* **189**: 278–87.

Riskind JH, Williams NL, Altman MD *et al.* (2004) Parental bonding, attachment, and development of the looming maladaptive style. *Journal of Cognitive Psychotherapy: an international quarterly* **18**: 43–52.

Rodebaugh TL, Holaway RM, Heimberg RG (2004) The treatment of social anxiety disorder. *Clinical Psychology Review* **24**: 883–908.

Rogers CR (1951) *Client Centred Psychotherapy*. Boston: Houghton-Mifflin.

Romme MAJ, Honig A, Noordhoorn EO *et al.* (1992) Coping with hearing voices, an emancipatory approach. *British Journal of Psychiatry* **160**: 99–103.

Romme MAJ and Escher S (1994) *Accepting Voices*. London: Mind.

Rosser RM, Birch S, Bond H, Denford J and Schachter J (1987) Five-year follow-up of patients treated with psychotherapy at the Cassel Hospital with nervous diseases. *Journal of the Royal Society of Medicine* **80**: 549–55.

Roth A and Fonagy P (2005) *What works for Whom?: a critical review of psychotherapy research* (2e). London: The Guilford Press.

Royal College of Psychiatrists (2002) *Requirements for Psychotherapy Training as Part of Basic Specialist Training*. www.rcpsych.ac.uk/PDF/ptBasic.pdf

Royal College of Psychiatrists (2005) *CBT Facts Sheet*. www.rcpsych.ac.uk/info/factsheets/pfaccog.asp (accessed 27 October 2006).

Ryle A (1995) *Cognitive Analytic Therapy: developments in theory and practice*. Chichester: John Wiley and Sons.

Safran JD and Segal ZV (1990) *Interpersonal Processes in Cognitive Therapy*. New York: Basic Books.

Salkovskis PM (1996) The cognitive approach to anxiety: threat beliefs, safety-seeking behaviour, and the special case of health anxiety and obsessions. In: Salkovis P (ed) *Frontiers of Cognitive Therapy* London: The Guilford Press, pp. 48–74.

Salkovskis PM, Jones DRO and Clark DM (1986) Respiratory control in the treatment of panic attacks: replication and extension with concurrent measurement of behaviour and pCO_2. *British Journal of Psychiatry* **148**: 526–32.

Salkovskis PM and Kirk J (1997) Obsessive-compulsive disorder. In: Clark DM and Fairburn CG (eds) *Science and Practice of Cognitive Behaviour Therapy*. Oxford: Oxford University Press, pp. 179–208.

Scher CD, Segal ZV and Ingram RE (2004) Beck's theory of depression: origins, empirical status, and future directions for cognitive vulnerability. In: Leahy R (ed) *Contemporary Cognitive Therapy*. New York: Guilford Press, pp. 27–44.

Scott J (2001) *Overcoming Mood Swings*. New York: New York University Press.

Scott J, Garland A and Moorhead S (2001) A pilot study of cognitive therapy in bipolar disorders. *Psychological Medicine* **31**: 459–67.

Scott J, Paykel E, Morriss R *et al.* (2006a) Cognitive-behavioural therapy for severe and recurrent bipolar disorders. Randomised controlled trial. *British Journal of Psychiatry* **188**: 313–20.

Scott J, Paykel E, Morriss R *et al.* (2006b) Cognitive-behavioural therapy for bipolar disorder [correspondence]. *British Journal of Psychiatry* **188**: 488–9.

Scott J, Stanton B, Garland A and Ferrier I (2000) Cognitive vulnerability in bipolar disorders. *Psychological Medicine* **30**: 467–72.

Segal ZV (1988) Appraisal of the self-schema constructs in cognitive models of depression. *Psychological Bulletin* **103**: 147–62.

Segal Z, Williams M and Teasdale J (2002) *Mindfulness-based cognitive therapy for depression: A new approach to preventing relapse.* New York: Guilford Press.

Sensky T, Turkington D, Kingdon D *et al.* (2000) A randomized controlled trial of cognitive behavioral therapy for persistent symptoms in schizophrenia resistant to medication. *Archives of General Psychiatry* **57**: 165–72.

Shapiro F (1995) *Eye Movement Desensitisation and Reprocessing: basic principles, protocols and procedures.* New York: Guilford Press.

Shapiro DA, Barkham M, Rees A *et al.* (1994) Effects of treatment duration and severity of depression on the effectiveness of cognitive-behavioural and psychodynamic-interpersonal psychotherapy. *Journal of Consulting and Clinical Psychology* **62**: 522–34.

Shapiro DA, Rees A, Barkham M *et al.* (1995) Effects of treatment duration and severity of depression on the maintenance of gains following cognitive-behavioural and psychodynamic-interpersonal psychotherapy. *Journal of Consulting and Clinical Psychology* **63**: 378–87.

Sharp DM, Power KG and Swanson V (2000) Reducing therapist contact in cognitive behaviour therapy for panic disorder and agoraphobia in primary care: global measures of outcome in a randomised controlled trial. *British Journal of General Practice* **12**: 963–8.

Shea MT, Elkin I, Imber SD *et al.* (1992) Course of depressive symptoms over follow-up: findings from the NIMH Treatment of Depression Collaborative Research Program. *Archives of General Psychiatry* **49**: 782–7.

Sijbrandij M, Olff M, Reitsma JB *et al.* (2006) Emotional or educational debriefing after psychological trauma: Randomised controlled trial. *British Journal of Psychiatry* **189**: 150–5.

Skinner BF (1950) Are theories of learning necessary? *Psychological Review* **57**: 193–216.

Smith JA and Tarrier N (1992) Prodromal symptoms in manic depressive psychosis. *Social Psychiatry and Psychiatric Epidemiology* **27**: 245–8.

Stangier U, Heidenreich T, Peitz M, Lauterbach W and Clark DM (2003) Cognitive therapy for social phobia: individual versus group treatment. *Behaviour Research and Therapy* **41**: 991–1007.

Stanley MA and Turner SM (1995) Current status of pharmacological and behavioral treatment of obsessive-compulsive disorder. *Behavior Therapy* **26**: 163–86.

Startup M, Jackson MC and Bendix S (2004) North Wales randomized controlled trial of cognitive behaviour therapy for acute schizophrenia spectrum disorders: outcomes at 6 and 12 months. *Psychological Medicine* **34**: 413–22.

Startup M, Jackson MC, Evans KE and Bendix S (2005) North Wales randomized controlled trial of cognitive behaviour therapy for acute schizophrenia spectrum disorders: two-year follow-up and economic evaluation. *Psychological Medicine* **35**: 1307–16.

Stone MH (1993) Long-term outcome in personality disorders. In: Tyrer P and Stein G (eds) *Personality Disorder Reviewed.* London: Gaskell, pp. 321–45.

Swartz M, Blazer D and Winfield I (1990) Estimating the prevalence of borderline personality disorder in the community. *Journal of Personality Disorders* **4**: 257–72.

Teasdale JD (1999) Emotional processing: three modes of mind and the prevention of relapse in depression. *Behaviour Research and Therapy,* **37**(suppl 1): S53–S78.

Teasdale JD and Barnard PJ (1993) *Affect, Cognition and Change.* Hove: Erlbaum.

Teasdale JD, Segal ZV, Williams JMG *et al.* (2000) Prevention of relapse/recurrence in major depression by mindfulness-based cognitive therapy. *Journal of Consulting and Clinical Psychology* **68**: 615–23.

Thase ME, Greenhouse JB, Frank E *et al.* (1997) Treatment of major depression with psychotherapy or psychotherapy-pharmacotherapy combinations. *Archives of General Psychiatry* **54**: 1009–15.

Thom A, Sartory G and Johren P (2000) Comparison between one-session psychological treatment and benzodiazepine in dental phobia. *Journal of Consulting and Clinical Psychology* **68**: 378–87.

Thompson LW, Coon, DW, Gallagher-Thompson D *et al.* (2001) Comparison of desipramine and cognitive/behavioral therapy in the treatment of elderly outpatients with mild-to-moderate depression. *American Journal of Geriatric Psychiatry* **9**: 225–40.

Thompson-Brenner H, Glass S and Westen D (2003) A multi-dimensional meta-analysis of psychotherapy for bulimia nervosa. *Clinical Psychology: Science and Practice,* **10**: 269–87.

Thorndyke EL (1898) Animal Intelligence. *Psychological Review Monograph Supplement* **2** (4, Whole No. 8).

Tien AY (1992) Distribution of hallucinations in the population. *Social Psychiatry and Psychiatric Epidemiology* **26**: 287–92.

Treasure J, Schmidt U, Troop N *et al.* (1996) Sequential treatment for bulimia nervosa incorporating a self-help manual. *British Journal of Psychiatry* **168**: 94–8.

Trinder H and Salkovskis PM (1994) Personally relevant intrusions outside the laboratory: Long-term suppression increases intrusion. *Behaviour Research and Therapy* **33**: 833–42.

Trull TJ, Nietzel MT and Main A (1988) The use of meta-analysis to assess the clinical significance of behaviour therapy for agoraphobia. *Behaviour Therapy* **19**: 527–38.

Turkington D, Kingdon D, Rathod S *et al.* (2006) Outcomes of an effectiveness trial of cognitive-behavioural intervention by mental health nurses in schizophrenia. *British Journal of Psychiatry* **189**: 36–40.

Turkington D, Kingdon D and Turner T (2002) Effectiveness of a brief cognitive-behavioural therapy intervention in the treatment of schizophrenia. *British Journal of Psychiatry* **180**: 523–7.

van Boeijen CA, van Oppen P, van Balkom AJ *et al.* (2005) Treatment of anxiety disorders in primary care practice: a randomised controlled trial. *British Journal of General Practice* **55**: 763–69.

van Etten ML and Taylor S (1998) Comparative efficacy of treatments for posttraumatic stress disorder: A meta-analysis. *Clinical Psychology and Psychotherapy* **5**: 126–45.

van Oppen P and Arntz A (1994) Cognitive therapy for obsessive-compulsive disorder. *Behaviour Research and Therapy* **31**: 79–86.

Vaughn C and Leff JP (1976) The influence of family and social factors on the course of schizophrenic illness. *British Journal of Psychiatry* **129**: 125–37.

Verheul R, van den Bosch L, Koeter M *et al.* (2003) Dialectical behaviour therapy for women with borderline personality disorder: 12-month, randomised clinical trial in the Netherlands. *British Journal of Psychiatry* **182**: 135–40.

Vitousek K (1996) The current status of cognitive-behavioural models of anorexia nervosa and bulimia nervosa. In: Salkovskis PM (ed) *Frontiers of Cognitive Therapy.* New York: Guilford Press, pp. 383–418.

Waddington L (2002) The therapy relationship in cognitive therapy: A review. *Behavioral and Cognitive Psychotherapy* **30**: 179–91.

Wampold BE and Messer SB (2002) Let's face facts: common factors are more potent than specific therapy ingredients. *Clinical Psychology – Science Practice* **9**: 21–5.

Ward E, King M, Lloyd M *et al.* (2000) Randomised controlled trial of non-directive counselling, cognitive-behaviour therapy, and usual general practitioner care for patients with depression: I. Clinical effectiveness. *British Medical Journal* **321**: 1383–8.

Watson JB (1930) *Behaviorism.* New York: WW Norton (reprinted 1970).

Wegner DM (1989) *White Bears and Other Unwanted Thoughts: suppression, obsession, and the psychology of mental control.* New York: Guilford Press.

Weissman AN and Beck AT (1978) Development and validation of the dysfunctional attitude scale. *Paper presented at the Annual Meeting of the Association for Advancement of Behavior Therapy,* Chicago, Illinois.